What others are saying about
Faces of Huntington's:

"In these pages, Carmen has captured the indomitable human spirit. *Faces of Huntington's* is a must read whether you are in a family affected by HD, a medical professional, or simply someone who cares."

Jim Pollard, Executive Director
Mediplex Rehabilitation and Skilled Nursing Center of Lowell

"*Faces of Huntington's* is a thoughtful, candid, brutally honest, excellent resource book. This thought provoking book is a great resource, and a source of comfort for anyone who is working with or has a chronic, terminal, or disabling disease. Eye opening from the employer perspective, *Faces of Huntington's* is a library must for an occupational health practitioner."

Terri Janda, RN BSN, Corporate Nurse Coordinator
Occupational Health Nurse Blue Cross Blue Shield of Kansas

"The stories and poetry in *Faces of Huntington's* describe issues and concerns that many families with HD face. This book will provide comfort, humor, and hope for those who care for people with HD. This book will also be useful to student and practicing health professionals who assist families in coping with the long term effects of Huntington's Disease."

Janet K. Williams, PhD, RN, CPNP, CGC
Associate Professor, The University of Iowa
Past-president, International Society of Nurses in Genetics

"*Faces of Huntington's* leads us out of the fray of misunderstanding and stigma of neuropsychiatric disease, and documents in parallel, the journey to hope and consolation in the fellowship of those familiar with and suffering from the disease. It generates the perspective of personal understanding and empathy for its readers, sustained by not a singular style but the determined voices of many. These writings challenge our own struggles and sensitively convey both the measure of humanity which is afflicted, and the courage of those afflicted."

Jeffrey I. Bennett, MD, Director
Neuropsychiatry Clinics and Consultation Psychiatric Services
Assistant Professor of Clinical Psychiatry
University of Chicago Hospital

"This book is about ordinary people living extraordinarily heroic lives. It is a book needed by all, especially those of us in medicine, who, for so long, this disease has forced to face our own uncomfortable impotence... forced us to face our own, personal defeat. Bravo to Carmen, author of more than a book, author of so much to so many."

Philip S. Backus, M.D.

"*Faces of Huntington's* is not just about people with Huntington's. It is about nearly all of us, and about chronic, catastrophic, and terminal illness which we have, are, or will encounter in our lifetimes."

Catherine Puhr, ARNP

Faces of Huntington's

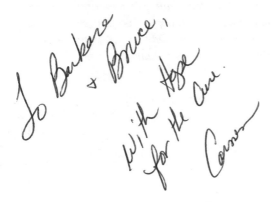

To Barbara & Bruce,
With Hope
for the Cure.
Carmen

Carmen Leal-Pock

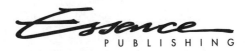
PUBLISHING

Belleville, Ontario, Canada

Faces of Huntington's

Copyright © 1998, Carmen Leal-Pock

ISBN: 1-894169-10-7

Cover illustration by Ruth Hargrave
Book Cover Design by Vickie Fraser

Essence Publishing is a Christian Book Publisher dedicated to further-ing the work of Christ through the written word. For more information, contact: 44 Moira Street West, Belleville, Ontario, Canada K8P 1S3. Phone: 1-800-238-6376. Fax: (613) 962-3055. Email: info@essence.on.ca Internet: www.essence.on.ca

Printed in Canada
by

Essence
PUBLISHING

I dedicate this book to my husband, Dave, who has Huntington's Disease. Without Dave, this book would never have been conceived of, or written. I also thank my wonderful sons, Nicholas and Justin, for being so special and helping me in ways of which they are not even aware.

$\sim$

This book is also dedicated to my brother Merrill. Though he didn't have Huntington's, Merrill fought his own battle with disease. Merrill's fight embodied much of what this book is all about. He fought the good fight with hope, faith, joy, love and so much more. I know, when he was done fighting, he was told, "Well done, good and faithful servant."

$\sim$

Lastly, this book is dedicated to all of the caring people in my life that helped me get to this point. You know who you are.

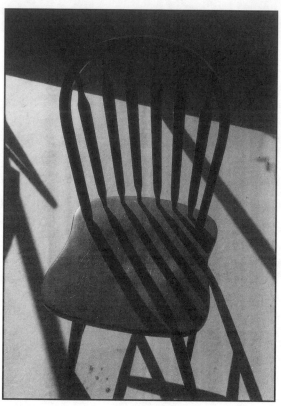

Photo: Nicholas Lucien Hahn

*For all those heroes of the Huntington's fight
who are no longer with us.*

*"I wanted a perfect ending. Now I've learned, the hard way, that
some poems don't rhyme, and some stories don't have a clear
beginning, middle, and end. Life is about not knowing, having
to change, taking the moment and making the best of it, without
knowing what's going to happen next. Delicious Ambiguity."*

—Gilda Radner

Contents

Acknowledgements

WRITING the dedication page of your book is a bit like accepting the Oscar for a hard earned Academy Award performance. You have so little space and so very many people to thank. I guess that's why the acknowledgment page was created – to thank all the people who helped to make the book a reality.

Without my Hunt-Dis family, this book might have been written, but it would not have been the rich, full one that it is. Thank you to this family that has been so much a part of my life for the last two years, and has seen me through each step of this insidious disease. Your openness, your willingness to help in any way you can, and your loving friendship, has often been what has gotten me through.

Again, the book might have been written without my gifted editor, but it would not have been quite as easy or wonderful. Thank you, JoAnn Zarling, for caring enough about the art of writing, myself, and thousands of people you don't even know, to help me create as fine a book as possible.

I remember when Dave was first diagnosed with Huntington's Disease. I went to my pastor and cried buckets of tears expecting him to tell me, somehow, that it would all go away and life would be normal. Darryl Keane did not try to make it better, but instead he said something I have thought of many times in the last three years. "I know you don't want to hear what I have to say. But I can see beyond where you are now. I can read the books you will write, hear the songs you will sing, and see the groups to which you will speak."

His statement did nothing to lift my wretchedness and I left the office feeling more bereft than I had ever felt in my life. On top of the sadness and grief, I was filled with anger. I did not want to see beyond where I was. I wanted to go back to where I had been before we learned the devastating news. Thank you, Darryl, for loving me enough to be honest. You knew I had been given the gifts of writing, singing, and speaking, and that at some point all of my life's experiences would come together for a purpose far larger than mine. They say no one is irreplaceable, but that simply isn't true. I miss you more than you can ever imagine. Thank you.

I have to thank my son Nick for bullying me into going on to the Internet when I thought it was a waste of time. Thanks to my technologically gifted son, I found information on Huntington's Disease, and a real family there as well. Nick also taught me how to create a web page and rarely laughed at me when I made mistakes. Nicholas and Justin both had to suffer the loss of their own computer time and the irritating tap, tap, tap of mother hunting and pecking late into the nights.

One evening, as I was chatting with a friend on the computer, we discussed my dream of writing a book for and about people with HD. This lovely man, who has a wife with HD, asked me what it would really take to get this book written. Sensing his sincerity, I told him I needed a new hard drive and a faster modem. Because I had so little space left on the computer, I could not write the book without a larger drive. Now, I won't mention his name or he would be deluged with requests for computer equipment, but "thank you" doesn't even begin to say what I mean. It wasn't just the modem and hard drive, it was that you believed in me, and were willing to spend money out of your own pocket to see this much-needed book be written.

There were so many people who sent me stories, quotes, ideas and good wishes, both through regular mail and E-mail. Obviously, there was no way I could use all that I received. Thank you to you who opened your lives to me. Much of this book was really written by those who cared enough to share. I just edited the submissions, and put them all together in what I hope is a readable format. In editing the many quotes, poems, and stories that make up this book, I worked to make only the minimum of changes. These changes in grammar and spelling were made to make what was being expressed more easily understood. The poetry in this book is written from the heart and was chosen to be included because of content, not perfection. I tried to retain the flavor of the pieces and for that reason, when you read this book, you will find different styles of writing.

Foreword

BY DR. RICHARD DUBINSKY

HUNTINGTON'S Disease was first described by George Huntington in the late 1800s. He had observed the disease when, as a boy, he made rounds with his father, on horseback, to visit the families that were affected by this illness. In his original report, he vividly described the choreaform (dance-like) movements, the problems with emotional control and thinking, and the inheritance from one generation to the next.

Over the last century, scientific knowledge of Huntington's disease has increased dramatically. The most striking finding in the brains of people who have died of Huntington's Disease is the loss of spiney neurons (nerve cells) in the caudate nucleus, a portion of the center of the brain. These neurons provide the connections between other nerve cells in the brain. Without these connections, we have difficulty in making everyday movements such as walking or eating. These connections are no different from our social connections that allow us to function in our society. Without them, we are isolated and clumsy.

We have known for many decades that Huntington's Disease was usually inherited from a parent who had Huntington's Disease, yet there were always cases where an affected parent could not be found. When Huntington's Disease was inherited from the father, the age of onset was earlier in the next generation, yet when inherited from the mother, it was about the same.

To better understand the inheritance of Huntington's Disease, a large scale study was undertaken in Venezuela, where Huntington's Disease is exceedingly common in the Lake Maricaibo region. In 1983, the genetic region for Huntington's Disease was found by this team. Ten years later they sequenced the gene and we could begin to understand the mechanisms of Huntington's Disease.

All of us have two copies of most of our genes, one inherited from our mother and one inherited from our father. We each have two copies of the INIT 15 gene, the gene that, when abnormal, causes Huntington's Disease. In Huntington's Disease, there is a stutter in the genetic code. The sequence CAG is repeated too many times, causing the protein made from the gene to be incorrect. At least three different mechanisms have been found where this abnormal gene product could cause Huntington's Disease.

The puzzling fact remains that the gene is abnormal from conception, yet the disease occurs only in the last one third of the person's life. This is also the same for those who contract the juvenile strain of Huntington's Disease, and those who have abnormally late onset. Though symptoms generally appear between thirty and fifty years of age, they have also appeared as young as two and as old as seventy, and progress over a ten to twenty-five year period. Based on these findings, the first multi-center studies of treatments, designed to slow the progression of Huntington's Disease, are currently underway.

Another outcome of the genetic research is the ability to tell if someone has the Huntington's Disease gene. In essence, a person can peer into their future to see if they will develop Huntington's Disease. The decision to undergo testing is a difficult decision to make and can have far-reaching consequences for the person and their family. Until a treatment is available that can slow the disease or delay the onset, pre-symptomatic testing will remain a very individual decision.

Despite all the research that has been completed and the studies still underway, Carmen's book reminds us that Huntington's Disease is not an entity in itself. It is a disease that affects people and their families and caregivers. Too often in the practice of medicine, we lose sight of the patient because of the disease. Clinicians and researchers, as well as caregivers and family members, need to be reminded that Huntington's Disease is an illness that affects people. The poignant and sometimes painful stories in *Faces of Huntington's* help us to catch a glimpse of the faces of those affected by this disease. By meeting the people in this book, we can learn lessons about Huntington's Disease that are as important as the research that has found the cause of Huntington's Disease.

Richard M. Dubinsky, M.D.
Department of Neurology
University of Kansas Medical Center

Preface

FACES *of Huntington's* is in no way a medical or scientific book. It is important to remember that there are no two people with this disease who have exactly the same symptoms in the same order. For instance, some people suffer with a tremendous amount of chorea, others barely have any. Additional symptoms may be equally different. The stories shared in this book are personal, and no one should project themselves or a loved one into any of the scenarios. This book is simply an honest look, through many eyes, of people who have and are living with HD.

In 1993, my husband was diagnosed with Huntington's Disease. We had never heard of HD, and when I went to the library in search of information, there was very little available. My first Huntington's convention in 1994 helped to a degree, but I still felt isolated by the lack of people who had HD in my area. I was also still frustrated that there was so little written for and about the people who daily fight the HD battle. In late 1994, my son introduced me to the Internet, and there I found more information than I had found in a year of searching bookshelves.

In this book, there are some terms that relate to the Internet. I use them almost without thinking now, because the Internet has become such a part of my life. Knowing there are many of you who are unfamiliar with this medium, several common internet terms are listed below.

For those who would like to know more about the available information on Huntington's Disease on the Internet, there is a reference section at the end of this book. I also recommend an excellent book called, *The Beginner's Illustrated Internet Directory*, by Betty Shulman. This easy to understand book will help you avoid becoming roadkill on the information superhighway. The book includes a wealth of basic knowledge about the Internet and should answer many of your questions. If you are interested in ordering this guide, call 1-800-444-2524.

Hunt-Dis is an on-line discussion group. This is a mailing list that allows individuals who are interested in all aspects of HD to communicate with each other. All you need in order to participate in a mailing list is E-mail access. E-mail stands for electronic mail. There are currently over three hundred people around the world on the Hunt-Dis.

The Internet is a vast network linking thousands of computers all over the world. These computers are physically connected to each other using special phone lines.

To explore all the Internet has to offer, you need to be on-line. When your computer establishes a connection through the modem, you are on-line and may begin using the various services on the Internet.

One last term used in a number of places in the book is pHD. This is a phrase that was coined on the Hunt-Dis as a form of short hand. pHD stands for "person with Huntington's Disease."

Carmen Leal-Pock

Introduction

Searching for a Cure II

BY GABRIELLE HAMILTON

Searching for a cure
    to save myself
from myself
    or inevitable betrayal
by the slow mutiny of
    my arms, legs and mind.

Searching for a cure
    while others hope
because I know what lays ahead
    and I have faith
in the dreams we've planned
    for tomorrow and ever after.

Searching for a cure
    so that your love for me

will not be spoiled
    by the monster
that is Huntington's Disease
    whose hold on me tightens
each year
    despite our valiant attempts
to remain at large.

Searching for a cure
    for others like me
who sometimes wish
    they'd never been born
to suffer
    this weighty burden.

January 12, 1996

If He's the One Who's Sick, Why Do I Feel Like Dying?

BY CARMEN LEAL-POCK

It was our third wedding anniversary. The day flew by at whirlwind speed as I went to work, shuttled the kids to and from soccer, cooked dinner and went about the daily routine. Having come out of a previous marriage fraught with anger, erratic schedules and a myriad of other problems, I focused on the wonderful solidity of my David. He did not have a charismatic personality nor would he ever earn substantial sums of money. But he adored me, was a hard worker, a romantic, and a strong Christian. I spent some of that anniversary day contemplating a long, secure marriage.

An hour after I thought David would be home from the doctor, he dragged himself into the house. The drawn look on his ghostly-pale face was only the first indication that something was extremely wrong. I tried to discover what had caused him to appear so much older now than he had just that morning. Without knowing what was wrong, I somehow understood the severity of the moment.

Instead of the joyous celebration, plans and gifts were abandoned as we began to discuss what we were facing. David seemed unable to articulate the diagnosis or even the thoughts churning in his mind. I was stunned by the news. My first response was to enfold my best friend in my arms as our separate thoughts became entwined. As the tears coursed down my face, everything within me silently screamed. Our anniversary was to be a time to celebrate our love, a time to plan for our future. The timing seemed a cruel hoax that I could not understand.

My sons bounded into the house, unaware of the tragic news, and we somehow went through a charade of our nightly routine. With the homework done and the chores completed, Nicholas and Justin prepared for bed. I silently begged for strength to get through prayer time with each son.

The nightmare of our anniversary finally ended and we sought refuge in each other's arms. Lying in bed, I knew one thing could not change. As angry as I was with this turn of events, I knew we had to continue to pray to God. I searched my mind for some praise to offer God as a way of starting off our nightly prayers. I thanked Him for three wonderful years of marriage, took a deep breath and somehow continued. After what seemed an eternity, I fell into an uneasy sleep.

I had never heard of Huntington's Disease, nor was I particularly knowledgeable about the brain in general. I began to search for information, thinking somehow that with knowledge there is power. I just knew that if I could talk to the professionals I could get a handle on this thing. We would spend every penny, make every sacrifice, if only Dave could be spared.

But no matter how much I wanted it to be different, there was no treatment and no cure. It seemed David had lived since birth with the time bomb of the gene which causes Huntington's Disease. Unknown to any of us, David's mother had been afflicted with Huntington's. As the facts became real, I learned this would be a long-term disease. I contacted the Huntington's group in New York and was soon inundated with information. I began to learn far more than I ever wanted to know.

The pieces of the puzzle that was Huntington's Disease slowly shifted into place, unasked questions were answered, and the completed picture became painfully clear. The constant movement wasn't nerves like I thought, it was HD. So was the forgetfulness, the indecipherable handwriting, the drunken walk, the slurred speech and innumerable other physical signs. The irrational anger that exploded unbidden, the numerous falls, and the poor way of handling finances were just three other signs. The list continued to grow until I was consumed with guilt that I had not forced him to see a doctor sooner. The deadly progression of HD had set up camp in his brain and nothing would persuade it to break ranks.

A series of bad falls had been the catalyst to seeing the doctor and to the ending of David's working days. Looking back, HD was probably the reason for his lack of assertiveness and, consequently, his halt midway in the climb up the corporate ladder. HD probably helped to end his previous twenty-one-year marriage. I know it affected his disciplinary skills along with his ability to get a new job.

At forty-three years of age, David shuffles through his days like an old man of eighty. As his appetite and ability to swallow continue to decrease, so does his weight. I am never sure who lives in his body. Is it my best friend? Or has the obstinate child who replaces David come to visit? His childlike tantrums coupled with his helplessness bring me to tears. Sometimes there is a violent person in his body, and at other times, it is an old man who sits and stares into space. Each of these people throws me into a turmoil that ends with a cry to God to please give me back my husband.

Every family who experiences the shock of HD reacts in a different way. HD is not only a disease of the afflicted; the entire family suffers. For my family, the challenges of step-parenting were thrown into disarray as David slowly lost control of his authority. I increased my work load at the office and at home. Ensuring that the car is in working condition is my total responsibility now that David no longer drives. That in itself is a problem because I have to run every errand and take the children to each school or sports event. The uncertainty of the future in terms of finances and how I will care for David is a panic which never leaves my mind.

The worse part of HD, for me, is losing my best friend in bits and pieces. I find myself erecting barriers around my heart to steel myself against the inevitable loss. Just when I persuade myself that the changes in David are permanent, he'll have a good day when he is close to being his old self. I fall in love with him all over again; then I watch him slip away. The grief that washes over me brings me to my knees to cry out my anguish to God once more.

Throughout this time, I have learned that as much as I love my husband, God loves Him even more. I know that there is a reason why we are being allowed the privilege to walk through this together, though daily seeing our suffering as a privilege is no easy task.

I have often asked, "Why must I suffer?" My suffering does a marvelous job of keeping me from pride. My suffering also is a constant reminder of just how much Christ suffered for me. What I am feeling is minuscule by comparison.

I am learning to understand that my suffering is only for a brief time when compared to eternity. There is a better time beyond earth. How I face my struggles is living proof of my faith in God. My struggles are not private. Both Christians and non-Christians are able to look into the fishbowl of my life and evaluate just how real God is to me. Finally, my struggles give God the opportunity to show His power.

Does my faith make me less vulnerable to those days all HD caregivers experience? Of course not. There are days I feel no one else can ever cry because I have used all their tears. What my faith does is give the assurance of God's promises that He will never leave me and He will provide for my every need.

When I compare my list of blessings against my concerns, the scale tips in the balance of blessings. On those occasions, when my grief blinds me to my blessings, God's strength is still sufficient for me. I keep remembering that I got through today and I will get through tomorrow. My job is to love and enjoy my husband. God's job is to take care of the details.

∽ 1

My Story

BY CARMEN LEAL-POCK

I WILL never forget the moment I first heard the words, "Huntington's Disease." Without even knowing what it meant, I knew it was bad. Worse than bad. After numerous falls at work, my wonderful husband of three brief years had been referred to a neurologist. I thought he was just clumsy, so I wasn't really worried. Until I saw his face.

It was September 28, 1994, our third anniversary. He was late, and I'd been working up a good bit of anger because we had dinner plans. I forgot all that when he told me the news. A few days later, we met with the neurologist and I learned I had good reason for my fears.

Dave's mother had been sick for quite a long time. I never met her and Dave had not seen her in years. By the time Dave was diagnosed, she had died. She had been adopted so there was no family history. When we were dating, Dave told me his mom was in Pennsylvania, remarried and sick with Multiple Sclerosis. I knew that was a horrible disease, but not genetic, so I didn't worry.

As I began to learn more about HD, and hear others' stories, I heard of this scenario quite often. A lack of family history and misdiagnosis is not uncommon.

I've heard many horror stories of those who went from doctor to doctor trying to find a reason for their behavior, or their falls, or their disjointed movements. With Dave, it was very simple. I am thankful we were members of an HMO. We ended up with a wonderful young neurologist who had finished her training in San Diego, working with a movement disorder clinic. Dr. Chiu knew Huntington's. She knew it well, and she knew Dave had it virtually the minute he walked into her office. But they went through the motions of determining if he had other diseases that would account for these symptoms anyway. I am sure Dr. Chiu would love to have been proven wrong, but she was right. Dave joined the elite group of people who have Huntington's Disease.

Dr. Chiu went on to tell us the truth. She didn't sugarcoat it or offer us false hopes. For this, I am grateful. She told us that HD is a devastating, degenerative brain disorder for which, right now, there is no cure. She outlined the course this disease would take and sent us on our way.

Dave had a good job when he lived in Phoenix. He'd been laid off due to an economic crunch, but we had no reason to believe he wouldn't be able to find employment again. Not long after he'd moved to Hawaii after his divorce, we met and married. Eventually, he got a job with the State of Hawaii, but it became clear after he started the job that in no way could he perform the duties of a Budget Analyst. I have to laugh now at the irony of a person in that stage of Huntington's being a number cruncher. It just wasn't funny at the time. Dave was tested and it was determined he was dyslexic. Under the Americans with Disabilities Act, his job was protected even though we now know he never had dyslexia. Because of the ADA laws, they couldn't let him go for poor job performance until they had made every reasonable effort to find him duties that he could perform. They could, however, shift him from job to job, trying to match his skills with a position. I believe that God really protected Dave as he was placed in the mail room and had to drive around the city of Honolulu. After a few fender benders and mail going to all the wrong places, Dave was transferred to the landscaping department. As much as he loved working in the gardens, it was probably the worst job they could have given him. Imagine a person with HD using power tools every day. Dave routinely fell into fish ponds and flower beds, and it was ultimately these falls that got him in to the neurologist. Despite the tools and falls, he was never badly injured.

After diagnosis, it was determined by his employers that they had fulfilled the "every reasonable effort" part of the ADA law. Though this was a financial blow to us, it was a relief to Dave. I look back and wonder how Dave managed to do physical labor in the hot Hawaiian sun every day. He was six foot four inches and had dropped to one hundred forty-six pounds.

Even though Dave had been working long enough to receive benefits, he had never passed probation. Moving from department to department had created the loophole the state needed and we were now without his income and medical benefits.

Again we were blessed. His files from the state, coupled with a well-written letter by Dr. Chiu, were enough to get Dave Social Security benefits within weeks of applying. I continue to hear horror stories of the social security system. I am so thankful that in our case we didn't have to go through all the red tape.

While Dave was going through his tests and dealing with HD, I was going through my own series of problems; I had to adjust to being married to a man I knew was dying. It became routine to play referee between Dave and my youngest son from a previous marriage. I had heard that a person with Huntington's often focuses on one person; Justin became the target for Dave's abuse and crazy behavior. Contrary to having a man who would act as a father figure to my sons, it seemed as if I now had three kids.

Dave did all types of crazy things with money. One time, I had a series of bouncing checks. I couldn't figure out why there was no money in the account until I finally pieced together this story. I used to make lunch for Dave and, as he had quite a sweet tooth, I always made sure there were cookies and desserts for him. It seems one brand of cookies I bought was popular in the office, so one day he went to the ATM, took out two-hundred dollars, then went to the store and bought cookies for his coworkers. His generosity resulted in our having to pay out hundreds of dollars in bank fees. Dave did so many odd things before his diagnosis, it made me wonder what had happened to the man I had married.

Before then, I had never heard of Huntington's Disease. One thing I know about myself is that I really don't like being around sick people. I remember the looks on the faces of people at church when Dave and I stood and asked for prayer. I was one of eight children and my mother did not have time for us to be sick. In fact, we were each allowed one sick day a year. My younger brother took this quite seriously. He asked mom since she was the mama, could she be sick for two days? Now, I asked those dear friends in the church to pray for Dave. But I also asked them to pray for me. I said something really sensitive like,

"Please pray I can handle this. I don't do sick. I always thought if you are sick, get drugs and get better. If that doesn't work, then please have the good grace to die." Of course, now that it was my husband who was sick, my opinion of illness changed. I would willingly nurse him no matter what. You can imagine how well that went over. But they got my point. I was in something I really felt ill equipped to handle.

Though people cared, they just did not "get it." People wanted to help, no one wanted to see me in pain. Sometimes the words that came out of their mouths were insensitive at best. My favorite was a friend at church who, a few weeks after diagnosis, walked over to me, looking aggrieved. She gave me a big hug. Trust me... she should have left it at that. She said, "I am so sorry to hear the news about David. But that's OK. When he dies, you will still be young and you can lose all your weight and get married again."

That was supposed to be a comfort? You have written off my husband, hastened his death, called me fat, and married me to who knows what kind of loser man all in one breath. I am not normally speechless. But mercifully for her, I was that day. There were many other comments but that was truly the jewel of them all. Thank goodness there were even a few helpful words given by others.

As the economy worsened in Hawaii, it became apparent that a move should seriously be considered. I was self-employed and losing my largest client while trying to hold the family together. The cost of living in Hawaii, and the lack of insurance made it impossible to live there. I was devastated. It was bad enough to be losing my husband to something I had never heard of. Now my children, who had never asked to get involved with this man, were going to have to leave their island home of fourteen years as well as their dad.

A long search led us to the Orlando, Florida area. Since moving, life has been a challenge. We are exhausted by the chase for Medicaid and Medicare benefits, and tens of thousands of dollars in debt. Dave was supposed to be my happily-ever-after. Things have turned out just a little differently than I had imagined they would when I promised to marry Dave for better or worse. This was much worse than anyone could have predicted. Certainly I had every right to walk away.

Living with HD is a lonely place to be. When we learned about Dave's illness, I rushed to the encyclopedia and found only a brief paragraph about it. I went to the library, and all I could find was medical jargon I could not and did not want to understand. *I wanted to know how to cope.* There was no support group in the islands and nothing written that I could find that would help. I did start a small support group in Hawaii, but the only other person with HD was a lady who lived in the hospital where the meeting was held. Everyone else was at-risk or positive and not symptomatic. There were no other caregivers.

Huntington's Disease Society of America did send me some helpful information about the disease itself and how to care for a person with HD. I also bought some excellent books. Yet nowhere did I read of people like me and how they were coping.

Nine months after diagnosis, Dave and I attended the annual HDSA convention in Pennsylvania. I was not prepared for the information overload and for seeing not one, but many persons with Huntington's. Before the convention, there was a call for writings relating to HD. I sent in a story and was selected to read my piece at the closing session. All the writings were emotional and the tears poured. Everyone in the audience was moved by the courage and love of those who read their stories. My piece was the last to be read.*

I had written about my impressions as a wife who has just heard about the disease. Tears filled my eyes and cascaded down my face making it difficult to read. The sounds of others crying made it all the more difficult, yet somehow I made my way to the end of the story. The silence in the hall was punctuated by sniffles and slight sounds, and then the applause began and swelled. The convention was officially over.

Making my way down the stairs, I was surrounded by people. "May I have a copy of your story? I want to give it to my counselor, my doctor, my wife, my pastor, my friends." People lined up to give me their addresses. What I had shared was not great writing. It was nothing unique. But I had managed to capture the essence of what others were feeling, and put it into words. People could identify with my feelings of hurt and anger and loss and fear. They wanted to be able to have something tangible to take and give to others and say, "Read this. This is how I feel."

When things get tough, I have to keep reminding myself of several things. This is not the first disaster I have faced, and it won't be the last. Others have survived worse, and I will survive this. Whatever doesn't kill me will make me stronger. Get the picture? I know that no matter how bad something is, something good can always come from it. Ralph Waldo Emerson said, "For everything you have missed, you have gained something else." I can honestly say I have lost much because of my association with Huntington's Disease. On the other

---

* "If He's the One Who's Sick, Then Why Do I Feel Like Dying?" appears on page 22.

hand, I have gained many things. I have met some of the most incredible people since we found out the news. These are people who have enriched my life as no one else. I have grown closer to God and have begun writing, which has opened many doors. I have become a stronger, more compassionate person, and have been able to reach out and support many people.

I could fill the next few hundred pages with all kinds of medical jargon and explanations. I could relive each painful ordeal my family has gone through because of HD. I could make you hate Huntington's as much as I do. I am not going to do that. This book is about the *people* side of HD. I can write about being a caregiver. I can't write, with authority, about being at-risk. Nor can I share about having HD, or having at-risk children. But I know people who can and will. This book is for those in the battle who want to find someone who knows what they are experiencing. We all need words to give to others and say, "This is how I feel."

In the past, I was a volunteer with the American Cancer Society. It wasn't that I had this great urge to see cancer eradicated, though that would be wonderful, of course. I did it because I had a friend who asked for my help. At a thank you ceremony for volunteers, the speaker asked a series of questions. He asked if there was anyone who was there because they were a cancer survivor. Were there any who had lost a spouse or a sibling or a relative? How about a coworker? With each question, more people stood until I was the only one sitting. I was shocked at all the people who had lost someone to cancer. At that moment, I realized that there were so many volunteers, such great sums of money donated, so much awareness of the problem, because cancer *has a face*. The faces of cancer to these and other volunteers are precious. The faces were forever burned in hearts, urging people to give of themselves until a cure can be found.

There are faces of Huntington's. But because there are so few compared to other diseases, some people have never seen a face of Huntington's or heard its voices. That doesn't change the fact there are faces.

It is my hope that *Faces of Huntington's* will be one catalyst to creating awareness, raising funds and someday finding a cure. Or maybe it will simply be a book that gives even one person hope. Either way, I would like to introduce you to some of the faces of Huntington's.

2

Faces of Encouragement

BY CARMEN LEAL-POCK

> T*here are no problems we cannot solve together, and very few that we can solve by ourselves.*
>
> —Lyndon Baines Johnson

Faces of Huntington's is not a medical book. It doesn't strive to delve deeply into the psychological aspect of this disease. Nor does it hope to answer every question you ever wanted to know about Huntington's. Instead, *Faces of Huntington's* is about people; people who just happen to be in some way associated with a devastating disease.

Have you ever gone to your son's or daughter's soccer game? Suppose you do, and there you see all the parents calmly sitting and watching, seemingly oblivious to the personal struggles and victories happening on the field. You see a spectacular play by your youngster and begin to clap and cheer. People stare at you as if you're not only an annoyance, but crazy as well. You have a choice. You can keep on applauding, knowing how positive this is for your child and the team, or you can quit. You choose to continue, and all of a sudden, another parent nearby begins to chant. Then another. And another. Finally, the once subdued field of spectators is filled with yelling, clapping and smiling parents.

It's a funny thing, in tandem with the cheering parents, the players are responding with renewed efforts. They are making goals never before thought possible. The frenzied pace of your cheering spurs them on to greater endeavors. You are making a difference; helping them win the game.

This book is about a group of people united by a common cause. Some of us are players, others are on the bench, still others are spectators. If I try to increase awareness of this disease by myself, I will be as effective as that one lone clapping parent. I have a caregiver's perspective. Others have shared their stories as persons with HD, or being at-risk, or caring for loved ones unselfishly, only to watch them deteriorate before their eyes.

Thank you to those who have decided to stand up and clap and cheer. Each time you share your story, each time you give someone something to read about Huntington's, you are a voice. Each time you explain to a member of the medical profession what this is all about, you are being heard. Every piece of red tape you cut through is a victory. Alone, we are scoring points. Together, we will win the game.

"The friend... who can tolerate not knowing, not curing, not healing and face with us the reality of our powerlessness, that is a friend who cares."
—Henri Nouwen

Even before each of us discovered the existence of Huntington's Disease in our families or ourselves, we needed support. That is how life is designed. Sometimes it is difficult to find encouragement when we need it. Whether it is because we are isolated physically or are trying to continue hiding the secret of HD, it's hard.

In the past, in so many families, HD was never discussed. Why would encouragement be needed if there was no disease? For years people have lived alone with the devastating effects of HD. In some ways, this is worse than the disease itself.

In a perfect world, there would be no HD, the term dysfunctional would not be applied to families, support groups wouldn't be needed, and no one would suffer, much less suffer alone. So much for a perfect world.

Support and encouragement comes in different forms. Natural families can and should offer tremendous support in coping with HD. However, support groups, church families, neighbors, and friends all have their place as well. Now with the advent of the Internet and computer prices dropping, support is often a click away. Support on-line comes in many forms. From a bulletin board to post and receive messages, to an E-mail distribution list, to actual real time chatting, support is there. A listing of Huntington's chapters and support groups, as well as directions for finding support on the Internet, can be found in the resource section of this book.

One of the members of an on-line group wrote, "I love all you people on this list because you are the support I never had growing up."

Another commented, "There is so much pain and so much love here. I don't feel I have much to say. Just a lot of whining. When you are alone, you feel you are the only family with this terrible disease." The National Huntington's Disease Society of America's motto is, "You Are Not Alone." Yes, there are others out there who are fighting the same battles, but without people to relate to, it's easy to feel alone.

After all the medical facts are digested and we become more expert on this disease than the doctors who treat HD patients, we are still the ones who have to live with it every day. Being part of a support system provides contacts with situations like yours. Sharing feelings, compassion, findings, laughter or tears does not mend hurting hearts, but it goes a long way towards enlarging those hearts. The common theme in any support group is growth, acceptance, understanding, and the ability to give and receive more love.

Receiving support from someone who has been or is in the same situation can often lead to useful advice. Something we say that seems like a random comment can be just what someone else needs to hear. My friend Ruth was saying just how much a friend had helped her put things into focus. Ruth's son has a twenty-five foot sailboat. He also has a problem with alcohol. Consequently, she seems to stay in a state of worry about his welfare. Oh, that worry may be warranted, but at this time, there is nothing she can do to change the situation. After hearing Ruth express her anguish over this son, her friend replied how she would give anything to see her own son with the desire to be independent.

Ruth admitted she had never looked at it in just that way. As a loving mother, she had only feared for his present safety, and not for his future. That one comment opened her eyes. Ruth stated what I have gone through so often myself. "I thought I had turned him over to God, but I guess I was trying to do God's job."

She is now trying to show more interest as he gets ready to live on the boat for the summer. All the worrying in the world won't change the fact that he is going to live on that boat and that he is extremely vulnerable. Ruth and her son can enjoy this time with each other instead of her existing in a constant state of panic.

We just don't know how our words and actions reach out to people. Sometimes we get in the rut of our own personalities and need another outlook at the same problem.

Regardless of what you may be feeling, whatever you are experiencing, another has been through it before, and another will go through it again. As the saying goes, "There is nothing new under the sun." Often we have no choice about what things we have to do, but we can always choose how we will do them. This goes for everything from the attitude we exhibit while doing something we would rather not be doing, to the actual hands-on mechanics of the chore. Learning how others have handled similar situations will suggest ideas to improve our own coping strategies.

For those who have HD, support groups can be extremely liberating. I remember when David and I attended our first convention. Until that point, we had never seen another person with HD. We saw others with his peculiar gait walking throughout the lobby the minute we entered the hotel. David had not wanted to attend the convention, but when he saw there were many that had the same symptoms, relief crossed his face. I realized that for David, this was a validation that he was not different. With validation came acceptance and hope.

Helping those with Huntington's to have the best quality of life possible is not simple, especially if your doctor or other health professional has not personally dealt with HD in the past. Who then can be your teacher?

How others have creatively handled smoking or driving and HD can save someone else hours of frustration, and possibly lives. Learning how to use tools for communication in the latter stages can help an entire family. Shared recipes that provide nutritious and safe meals for one with swallowing problems make a world of difference to both the affected person and the caregiver. The list is endless on what we can learn from or share with others.

What we see as commonplace can be a breath of fresh air to another. One woman who had been isolated for many years recently found the on-line support group. She wrote, "I took care of my husband for thirteen years before he died and I felt so alone on this earth. Even close friends that knew of the situation just couldn't understand. It is a disease from hell. The person suffers from it and so do the caregivers. It feels so good to have someone ask me how I am doing. A big thanks. You made my day."

Such a little thing it seems, being asked how she was doing. For years this woman chose to be a caregiver. She spent over a decade answering the question, "How is your husband?" As valid a question as that obviously was, she was seldom asked the simple question, "How are you?" Everyone needs to know they have value. Three little words gave her value and still help her as she continues her caregiving since she also has children who are affected. The difference is, she now has found support to help along the way.

If you live in an area with an organized chapter or support group, consider becoming involved in their activities. What you can give is equally as important as what you receive. If there is not a group, consider starting one. You will find those who have a need to communicate with others in the HD community. And if you have a computer and a modem, on-line support can help fill the gap you may be feeling.

This Net
BY LEON JOFFE

Stranded I reach to clutch each strand of hope
To find a hand to touch that I may cope
With every moment's pain, though hidden deep
In work or chores or quiet or talk or sleep.

Lost I search the sea, the land, the air
The moon and stars themselves for those who keep
A secret song of love amid despair.
Before this, answers came but none to share.

For who but those who know can weave the rope
To pull me from madness; and who but those who care
Can teach me still to smile before I weep?

∽

It's the Little Things
BY SUSAN GARRETT

When I tell people I have tested positive for the Huntington's gene, I can see they feel badly and don't know what to say. If they really know about the horrors of this disease, I sense they are thinking about how I will be in the future.

Yes, I am HD positive and I am in the early stages. This morning I went for a checkup. We talked a lot about my loss of balance, and my doctor suggested I retire all of my high heels, as I am a serious accident waiting to happen. He said that is the last thing I should have to worry about.

I wear heels every day of the week, because they make me feel feminine. Stupid thing to be upset about I know, but it's just one more thing. I know it's a little thing, but that's what life is; groupings of little things that make us who we are. For me, the loss of my heels is much more than wearing flat shoes that don't make me feel feminine. It's just one more thing in a long string of future losses.

I was on Hunt-Dis one day and mentioned the loss of my heels. Instead of laughing at me, a friend from the list said, "The same thing happened to my wife years ago. Just yesterday, I found a pair of shoes in her possessions; they're shiny black and have very high heels. I remember seeing her in those heels some twenty years ago and thinking, 'Gosh, what a babe!' Now she is bedridden in a nursing home. In my mind, I see her in those heels and we're still walking together."

If I've lost my heels, I've gained friends and gotten support from people who have shown, in many ways, how much they care.

My friend at work, Chris, reacted this way to my flat shoes. "It's so hard to know how to act, speak, and feel, knowing that while for all of us marching through these halls, sitting in our cubes, it's just another day on the farm. But for you, every day is a reminder of what lurks ahead; no reprieve and no escape from the ever-present knowledge. I see you and act like everything is normal. For you, though, nothing will ever be normal again; or rather, there is a new and terrifyingly real normal."

He continued saying, "I want you to know that for me, you are a great example, and a reminder of what it means to be courageous. I cannot express the depth of my admiration for you. For as long as I've known you, I've perceived you as a person of great innocence, without guile, struggling through life's challenges as a single working mom, carrying more load than you deserve. To have this added on to you and to still function is amazing. Susan, the power of simple perseverance which you demonstrate daily is mind boggling. It speaks volumes about your power of spirit and depth of character, in spite of how insecure you might, or must feel. In fact, it is this ability to act in the face of insecurity that tells me of the inner strength and faith you have, whether or not you realize it.

"I want you to know that your heels will never define your femininity, but of course you know that. It's always your eyes I see, not your heels. I love who you are, Susan, and I want you to know that you are in my prayers. No matter what happens in this life, I have a testimony of the richness of your reward in the life to come, if you will continue to step into the shadows, despite your fear of the dark."

I miss many little things that I am gradually losing, and I know there will be more in the days and years to come. If I have to choose between the loss of those little things, and having such supportive and wonderful friends, I'll take the friends.

∽

The City

BY KEN SHEARS

I always smile when someone wanders into Hunt-Dis by mistake. I imagine them as medieval travelers entering a city where a peculiar plague has taken hold. The visitor senses that a great silent number may be holed up in their houses. They can see those who are helping the sick, and there are people in various stages of this odd malady walking the streets.

Some are very sick and cannot speak, while others show no signs of impending illness. For as many as wear haunted expressions of fear and grief, there are those who smile openly. The traveler even hears laughter leavening the solemnity and horror of what swirls around them. In a quiet corner someone weeps for their loved ones, for themselves. People rush to them, to comfort and lift them up.

In this city are scholars and doctors, working so intensely to discover the cause and a cure for the plague, that they sometimes buckle under the strain. There are writers and poets, clerics and scientists. This assortment of just plain folk are all focused on one thing – the afflicted. Whether they are about to embrace death, or just beginning to show signs, the concern is there.

Here and there are small groups talking to one another and the visitor hears snatches of their conversations. Some are so normal, small talk actually. The talk is of no consequence, but hearing it here in this city, it sounds abnormal. These are greetings amidst despair, salutations rising above heart felt prayers and lonely cries.

In this city, there are differences of opinion, sometimes sharp. Of course, it is understandable really. How is it that any of these citizens of this strange place cope? The visitor is struck most by how much the people know of their suffering; how well they help each other understand what is happening.

There is great hope in this city alongside great sickness of heart. Eventually, the traveler apologizes for coming, they are not from here, this place was not their destination, they turn and go. Later, they will tell others of the strange city where there was a plague, but where people could still laugh and openly converse. They cared for one another amidst great hardship and travail, and life in all its wonderful variety warred with death, where even disagreements led to healing. Maybe the traveler sees what a miraculous place it was they had visited, the city of Hunt-Dis@ Maelstrom.

How to Get to the City of Hunt-Dis@Maelstrom

A mailing list devoted to Huntington's Disease was started by Storm King, a graduate student in psychology at St. John's University, in March 1996. As of July 1997, there were over two hundred and fifty members with more being added almost daily.

The members of the list have a common interest in HD. Some have HD, some have tested positive, some are at-risk, some are caregivers, and some are doctors or genetics counselors. They are a wonderful group of people, all trying to help each other with information and support.

Often called on-line discussion groups, mailing lists allow individuals who are interested in similar topics to communicate with each other. To participate in a mailing list, you first must have a computer, a modem, and an E-mail address. Then you must subscribe to the list by sending a special command to the computer where the list is maintained. Once you are signed on, you can send messages and they will automatically be distributed to everyone else on the list.

You subscribe to the list by sending an E-mail message. You will then get a message back telling you that your subscription has been received, and asking you to send a confirmation to make sure your E-mail address works okay. After you reply to that message, you will get a message telling you your subscription has been accepted and giving you instructions on how to send messages to the list, how to set various options, and how to unsubscribe from the list. After that, you can send messages and you will receive, through E-mail, copies of all messages which are posted to the list, including your own.

Because privacy can be an issue for many people, if you don't want anyone to know you are on this mailing list, you can send a conceal command which will keep your name from showing on the list of subscribers.

To subscribe to the Huntington's Disease mailing list, send an email message to:
listserv@maelstrom.stjohns.edu
Leave the subject line blank.

In the body of the mail message, type the following:
subscribe hunt-dis yourfirstname yourlastname

Substitute your first name and your last name for yourfirstname and yourlastname above. It doesn't matter whether you use upper case or lower case in the body of the message.

Do not type anything else in the body of the message.

Send the message and in a few minutes you should get a reply back.

To get off hunt-dis, send a message to:
listserv@maelstrom.stjohns.edu

Leave the subject line blank.
In the body of the message, type:
signoff hunt-dis

Don't put anything else in the message.
Be sure you send the message to:
listserv instead of to hunt-dis.

This discussion list can be a great way for those who are concerned about Huntington's Disease to ask questions, share their ideas, and learn from each other. Please understand, the volume of the list is quite high and the messages varied. If you have only a limited amount of time to invest in a discussion of Huntington's Disease, you might wish to join a real time chat group or go to the many available web sites listed in the resource section of this book.

∽

Symphony of Unity
BY HAROLD

They told me
The world was lost –
Hopelessly divided and torn apart
By the passions of cruel men;
By evil men who spoke alien tongues,
Who would never understand
One another's wants.

I looked out
On the world around
And saw men of many nations and climes
Speaking many strange languages;
With manners and customs of many kinds.
Opinions and beliefs,
Principles and doctrines.

And I said,
"Yes, it is true.
Man is helplessly divided and torn apart
By a generation of cruel men –
By evil men who can only speak evil
Of one another,
And another's wants."

But then I heard
On a still night

A great symphony of instruments playing,
With delicate scales and rhythms,
With sweeping, massive chords and harmonies,
A moving hymn
And a quiet cadence.
I knew what it was –
A Bach chorale.
And it spoke to me a word of kindness,
I thought of comfort and encouragement.
I knew that men everywhere could hear it –
And hearing, understand
Its moving message.

It could have been
Any other chorus,
Or any other composer's creative masterpiece:
A Gregorian chant, a Tallis madrigal,
A Handel oratorio, A Beethoven symphony,
Or Aaron Copeland,
Or Shostakovitch.

The notes we know
And knowing, comprehend:
Whether they come from Germany or France
Or China or Israel, Poland, or Greece
Or Scotland or Italy, Russia or Sweden,
England, Hungary,
Or the Americas.

They speak as one –
A Universal language:
A grand tone-poem with a melodious leit-motif
Of unity close binding all the tribes of men:
Of harmony beneath the surface of clattering dissonance

FACES OF HUNTINGTON'S

Man's one-ness
With fellow-man.

And over all –
The God of all.
Eternal Father – called by many Names.
He has made of one blood all the nations:
One race – the living human race –
One universal lineage
Under Almighty God.

And Then There Were Two

BY SHIRLEY PROCELL

First there was one
Then there were two
I looked up at heaven
Said, "What will I do?"

I waited and waited
It seemed like for days
The answer was coming
God said, "There are ways."

Things I will teach you
Of patience and love
Things that will come
From heaven above.

Yes, He had the answers
How could I doubt?
He taught me through HD
What life's all about.
He gave me some friends
That are loving and strong
He told me to go there
When things go wrong.

Yes, first there was one
Then there were two
I no longer ask,
"What will I do?"

Untitled

BY GABRIELLE HAMILTON

You asked me
   how I feel
Unsure
   of what you could do to
help me,
   but
wanting desperately
   to do something.

You asked me
   how I feel
Scared
   that one day you would not
recognize
   my voice, my arms, or my face
as the ones
   you've always known.

You asked me
   how I feel
Hoping
   to prop me up

and give me
   strength for the long,
long battle ahead.

You asked me
   how I feel
Longing
   for someone to
strengthen you
   as you are
strengthening me.

And because of
   all of this
you know that
   when you ask me
how I feel,
   I am afraid.

February 28, 1995

3

Kym's Story

BY KYM NICHOLSON

C HRISTOPHER Dougles Youngblood was to be my awakening. I was very young, certainly not ready for a child. At the same time, I was excited about becoming a mommy.

We were told the disease that plagued my ex-husband's family was not to be worried about. It was an adult disease. If my son did happen to be afflicted with the defective gene, there would certainly be a cure by the time he was in his prime and beginning to show symptoms. This was our first clash with medical theories. I could never have imagined the events that would later unfold. They would change my life forever, in a way that no one's life should be lived.

Christopher was born on a beautiful, sunny spring afternoon. He was absolutely beautiful, and perfect in every way. He weighed in at seven pounds, two ounces and was nineteen inches long. He was also bald as a cue ball!

We were certainly the proud parents, probably patented the phrase. Everything was great for about a year. Then

Chris's dad and I started to part ways and Chris and I moved back home to Illinois to begin our new life together. I was pregnant and his sister was due a few weeks later. It was just him and me against the world.

It was tough. I was a very young mother with two babies, barely a year apart. I did not have enough education to support a family. By the age of three, Chris's speech became slurred, and his gait was unsteady. He seemed to be such a klutz! It didn't take long for me to figure out what the problem was, but the specialists certainly took what seemed like forever.

We had lived with my husband's family for the first seven months of our marriage. I had seen my ex-mother-in-law suffer the wrath of Huntington's Disease. I knew what was happening. What I didn't know was how much time I would have with my son. Christopher led a pretty normal life for almost seven years. After that, little by little, everything that gave him independence was slowly stripped away. At first, it was the speech, initially becoming slurred, then impossible for him to form the words.

We took sign language classes to help keep the lines of communication open for him and for us. Then the fine motor skills began to deteriorate. As this affected his signing, he was losing all means of communication. His gross motor skills were also diminishing, but thankfully, at a slower rate.

By the time he was seven years old, it was next to impossible to understand much of anything he was saying. By age eight and a half, his sign language had suffered as well. We could only communicate basic needs... eat, drink, toilet. Then, at age ten and a half, he took his final steps, and never walked again.

Christopher was always happy, with a wonderful disposition. He absolutely loved people, life, and his family.

There wasn't a person he met that wasn't somehow touched more deeply than they had ever been by another child. Everyone adored him. The kids at school would compete with each other to be there for Chris. They all wanted to push Chris' wheelchair, help feed him, refill his water bottle, and write his work for him. The bonds that he had woven with his friends, the love that he instilled through everyone that he encountered, and the mutual respect and admiration that everyone had for him were his reasons for living.

Throughout all the changes that occurred over the years, I was never prepared for what happened on February 7, 1997. It all started with a trip home to Illinois to visit his grandmother. Chris had not been feeling well that day, and was having sporadic movements in his left leg. These were movements that made his leg shoot straight up in the air, and then shoot back in a bent position. It happened in such a way that his knee would hit him, like a punch in the face.

Chris had zero reflexes with which to protect himself. When his leg would hit his face, he would scream in pain. No matter how many times we would hold his leg, massage it, or soak him in a warm tub, the movements refused to cease.

By the next evening, Chris was literally exhausted. He'd had no sleep for two days and was absolutely miserable, bordering on delirious. His temperature shot up to 104° F. He was admitted after we took him to the emergency room and immediately put on injections of Haldol through his IV unit.

I had gone to school to become a medical assistant. I had devoured every piece of information on Huntington's Disease, and all pharmacology information on every drug that was being used to treat this disorder. I was terrified of

Haldol, but I had seen all the suffering that Chris had endured the past two days and was willing to try just about anything.

The following morning, his neurologist came in to examine Chris, and then called me to a private family area. I knew what was coming before we ever entered that room. He proceeded to inform me that it was very important that I start making some decisions about Chris' treatment. Did I want him resuscitated should he arrest? How invasive did I wish the staff to be? Just how far did I want to take this?

I thought I was going to break. Nothing had ever hurt so much in my life. And who was I to play God, and choose whether my son should live or die, and when?

I came to the decision that if Chris should happen to stop breathing, I didn't want any heroic measures taken, and that he was not to be resuscitated. I justified this with the fact that if God allowed it to happen in the first place, it must be His will. That, and the fact that I couldn't bear to see him suffer needlessly. Huntington's Disease is relentless. It doesn't stop, get better, or give any hope. It only takes from the brain, muscular and nervous system, until there is nothing left to feed off. There is no treatment and no cure.

After two days of the Haldol, Chris was completely unresponsive and I refused another dose. I insisted upon valium. I knew that valium was very risky, due to the respiratory problems that can surface when used in children. I also believed it was the lesser of the two evils. After three doses, Chris calmed down. His leg stopped moving, and finally, he slept. He slept for hours and hours. I became uneasy, but convinced myself it was because of the lack of sleep over the last three and a half days.

My mother had come to the hospital to relieve me for

a few hours. Normally, it was Mom who held the bedside vigils with Chris. She was absolutely in love with him. They had such a special bond, it did not surprise me that he waited for her to be there before he awoke. I had been gone for about an hour when the phone rang and my mom told me to get back up there. Something had happened, and it was good. I flew! I don't know that the car's wheels ever really hit the ground at all. I do know that I made that twelve .minute trip in under six.

When I walked into the room, I was immediately in shock. I was seeing it, but somehow, my heart wouldn't let me believe it. Chris was sitting up, propped up on pillows, and smiling. His color was great, and he was completely alert and responsive.

I immediately said a heartfelt, "Thank you" to God, and burst into tears. Nothing has ever given me such joy and utter elation in my life. At the same time, I was scared to death. I was so afraid that this was just a fluke. I didn't want to hang my hopes just yet. I've never been a pessimist, but after seeing Chris so close to death earlier that day, I just didn't know what to expect.

Two days later, we took him home. Hospice was called in before we left the hospital, and had a hospital bed and all of his medications, syringes, and supplies delivered within an hour of our arrival. They became a big part of our lives from there on out. And they were wonderful. The day after we brought Chris home, the movements started again, and we battled to keep them under control. Chris was on a pureed diet and didn't have much appetite. He did, however, drink liquids by the masses, as he kept dehydrating from over-exertion. This went on for almost two weeks.

We bought a house, knowing we could not go back home to Michigan, and arranged to move our things. On

February 22, 1997, I began hauling our things down. On February 23, we brought Chris to his new home. That day was a very good day for Chris. He had very little movement in his leg and watched his cartoons all day. We stayed busy unpacking everything. However, he had drunk only two ounces of water all day, and wouldn't take anything else. That night, he started having movements again, and was moaning in his sleep.

At seven the next morning, I went into his room to give him his medications, and immediately froze. He was so pale, almost gray, barely breathing, and his nail beds were dark gray. I was horrified, and scared to death. I went to pick him up, and his bed and pillow were saturated with sweat.

By eight o'clock, I had him in the E.R. again. By 3:00 that afternoon, he was looking more normal, and I decided that I would take him home. I brought an extra IV bag with me for the next day. Deep inside, however, I knew that I would never use it.

I laid him in my bed and talked to him all night. He didn't appear to be with me, but there was a slight chance that he could still hear. I wanted him to know that I was there with him, and would not leave him. I told him to watch for the angels. They were coming, and when they did, it was okay for him to go with them. They would show him beautiful places, where he could run and talk and play, and he would never hurt or be sick again. He would go to a place where he would always be happy and be able to fly.

Chris took his final breath at 9:15 on Tuesday, February 25, 1997. How appropriate that he would wait until it was just his grandmother and me there with him – the two constants in his life who had always been there through everything that he experienced, good and bad.

I do not mourn his passing, only my loss and the empty space that he once filled so perfectly. Chris can now do all the things that were taken from him on this earth. He can walk, talk, run, play, laugh and fly.

I realize now that Chris was my angel. He was sent to teach me about what true love, compassion, and patience is all about. He truly was the very essence of love. He instilled in me an appreciation for life that I would never have acquired any other way.

Christopher is my idol, my mentor, my life's greatest love, and my rock. I can do anything, just knowing that his spirit is always here to guide, love, and comfort me. Heaven has been graced, and I have been blessed immeasurably. God has given me the greatest gift of all. The privilege of knowing real love, the honor of having Chris for those few wonderful, but short years.

∽ 4

Faces of Love

BY CARMEN LEAL-POCK

It is possible to give without loving, but it is impossible to love without giving.

—Richard Braunstein

Two of the most quoted passages from the Bible are about love. If you're a fan of professional football games, you've seen a parade of people over the years holding a simple sign. John 3:16 says, "For God so loved the world that He gave His one and only Son, that whoever believes in Him might not perish, but have eternal life." Whether you believe it or not, you have to admit that is love. For God to give His most prized possession for mankind? That is love.

I once heard a story of a young boy who had recovered from a rare disease. Two years later, his sister contracted the same disorder. Because of the rarity of their blood types and the disease involved, her only chance for survival was a transfusion of her brother's blood. When the doctor asked the boy if he would give blood to his sister, he said, "Yes." The day of the transfusion, the little boy was frightened. But it was for his sister; he could do this. When they were just about finished, the youngster looked up with huge eyes and said, "When will I die?" You see, the little boy believed that the procedure, while saving his sister's life, would rob him of his own. He loved his sister enough to give his life, his most precious possession, for her. That is love.

The second often quoted Bible reference is commonly called the "Love chapter." It is part of countless wedding ceremonies each year. 1 Corinthians 13:4-7 says, "Love is patient, love is kind. It does not envy, it does not boast, it is not proud. It is not rude, it is not self-seeking, it is not easily angered, it keeps no record of wrongs. Love does not delight in evil but rejoices with the truth. It always protects, always trusts, always hopes, always perseveres. Love never fails."

Boy, talk about some big shoes to fill! When I read that verse, I can only think of how short I fall of reaching the mark. Maybe that is why they say love is a process. But whether we are talking about romantic love, or love for a family member or friend, love is as important to those of us involved with Huntington's Disease as it is to anyone else.

The first person I met with Huntington's Disease, after my husband was diagnosed, was a woman named Margaret. When I met Margaret, a Canadian, she'd been living in a hospital in Hawaii for three or four years. I never heard all the bits and pieces of the story, but it seems while on vacation in the islands, Margaret got sick. She was hospitalized and has never left. Her family and friends live in Canada and have, as far as I can tell, abandoned her.

I'm sure Margaret had many people over the years say, "I love you." You can see remnants of her once elegant beauty. Her smile is still vibrant and personality shines through her eyes. Margaret cannot feed herself, or walk, or talk. She is dependent on the hospital staff for all her needs. Dave and I were her first non-medical visitors. The day I saw Margaret I knew, no matter what, I would be there for Dave. For as long as we lived in Hawaii, we visited Margaret at the hospital and she came to our support group meetings. Those monthly outings became the highlight of her existence. I am glad we were there for her, but I often wonder, is someone there for her now?

Living by the definition of love found in 1 Corinthians is hard even when things are going well. We are constantly falling short of self-expectation and then trying to improve. But when an illness as devastating as HD takes over our lives, the real challenge begins.

Lloyd is a special person; a caregiver who is committed to his wife, Joan. Lloyd has this to say. "I am determined to make Joan's progress through this disease as painless as possible by being there for her, and accommodating her in any way I can. That doesn't mean I don't get short-tempered and depressed at times. It's no picnic, but I am determined to see it through. It never fails to amaze me when acquaintances seem to suggest this is somehow odd or heroic. Why is that? I'm not the one suffering the ravages of Huntington's."

Yet compared to some of the trials and tribulations Lloyd sees for others who are involved with HD, he somehow feels lucky. He has his health and had just taken early retirement before they even found out about Joan having HD. They don't have children so the disease has not been passed on. He has the time and ability to look after Joan at home, so he is going to do it. "I don't see it as an obligation," he said. "I just believe it is the decent and right thing to do. I know Joan would do the same for me if the tables were turned." That is love.

Sometimes, depending upon the situation and the behavior exhibited with HD, the most loving thing to be done for yourself, your children and yes, the one with HD, is to not be together. I've heard countless stories of people who, given all the facts and after looking at all the options, have found divorce, separation, or a nursing home, to be the best arrangement. In many cases, the person with HD is still cared for by their family or visited in the nursing home. People are quick to make judgments and have strong opinions. If HD has taught me one thing, it is that I need to be there for those that need me, but not to make judgments. Each family is unique and has unique needs, and they have their own ways of dealing with it.

Jerry said, "The happiest day of my life was when I married Peggy thirty years ago. The saddest day of my life was January of this year, when I put her in a nursing home."

Jerry still adores his bride of thirty years even with the inevitable changes that come with Huntington's. He makes sure all her needs are met, and when there is a problem the nursing home can't solve, Jerry brings his questions to the on-line support group. Jerry sent a question to us about a health problem not related to HD. Peggy had what he later found out was a urinary tract infection. He posted questions to the list about causes and solutions for this problem. Many people were helpful in pointing him in the right direction to get his wife the help she needed. After it was resolved he posted this message.

"Funny, but I was less embarrassed posting to this list with hundreds of readers than I was buying the personal care products for Peggy. I learned more about feminine hygiene than I wanted to or should know. We caregivers do our very best for our pHDs. I made it through the blushing young girl at the drug counter. We were both bright red. Next was the charge nurse. I should have talked to her in private because I collected a large group of nurses and aides. The young aides blushed and I could see the nurses struggling to control their laughter. One nurse lost it and everyone started laughing. I felt like I was going to collapse so I left for my car. A nurse caught me just outside the building. She said, 'Jerry, please excuse us. It's just that we have never had such a pathetic lecture on feminine hygiene.' She took my sack of care products and said, 'We can handle it from here. You have made our day.' Any guy that tries to become an expert in feminine hygiene, and a sketch artist in an hour, and then winds up addressing a group of nurses, is a sick puppy. Now does anyone have any suggestions how I can improve my reputation with the nurses?"

I sat at my computer with tears streaming down my face as I pictured this dear man risking the embarrassment that would send most men into shock to help his wife. This too is love.

There are many kinds of love, but none so inspiring to me as the love a mother has for her child. As a mother, I have stood by helplessly as other children ignore my sons, or make fun of them for some perceived minor flaw. My heart aches for the hurt they feel. I am thankful I will never know the pain of seeing my children with Huntington's. Oh, they may have other illnesses and injuries over the years, but not HD.

Jean showed just how much she loves her daughter Kelly with a T-shirt they had made for her to wear in a large group of people. The front of the T-shirt said:

I have Huntington's Disease,
What's YOUR problem?

On the back, inside a broken heart was this poem:

To have someone stare so rudely
and assume that I am drunk or high,
hurts my very being
and causes my soul to cry.
So before you make judgements,
pointing or whispering callous names,
just remember someone is keeping score
and one day YOU'LL feel the shame.

Some people, in just seeing the front of the T-shirt, realized it was a disease and she wasn't high or drunk, and would look away. Some asked what Huntington's was. Most continued to be out-and-out rude, even after reading the back of her shirt. To those Jean responded, loudly, "Here but for the grace of God go you," or "It's obvious your mother never taught you any manners." Sometimes Jean felt such anger and would get so upset, but Kelly would say, "Mom, it's their problem, let it go." If it weren't for her, Jean says she probably would have decked most of them and be writing from jail. I have no doubt Jean would willingly go to jail if it would help Kelly in some way. The creativity Jean showed in creating such a T-shirt and standing by Kelly, no matter what, is incredible. Of course, beyond that, it is love.

It isn't only families that can show their love or desert a family with HD. One statement that caregivers continually make is about the sadness they experience when friends stop coming around after diagnosis. Shirley Procell has written two poems that say everything about this and more. She wrote these after getting home from work one day. Both of her sons with Huntington's were sitting on the porch hoping for a visit from a friend or, in her son Gary's case, one of his three children. The visitors never came.

∽

The Tears Never Dry

BY SHIRLEY PROCELL

> *He sits there alone*
> *Just watching T.V.*
> *Hopes for a call*
> *From one of his three.*
> *But the phone does not ring*
> *And the tears never dry*
> *It looks like just one*
> *Could call or drop by.*
> *He knows when you're young*
> *That you tend to forget*
> *That somewhere, someone*
> *Waits for you yet.*
> *It would take such a little*
> *To dry up those tears*
> *And give him some comfort*
> *He's not had in years.*

The Porch

BY SHIRLEY PROCELL

I glanced out my window
It was pouring down rain
Looked at the little house
That's so filled with pain.
On the porch, Ken was walking
In his stiff gaited way
Hoping a good friend
Might visit today
For his is a lonely life
Without very much hope
A visit is one thing
That helps him to cope
But people are busy
They don't understand
What one little visit is
To the soul of a man
So if you get bored
And need something to do
He has a porch
That is waiting for you
And on it's a man
That can't call out your name
But he'll be so grateful
And glad that you came.

Then there are friends that do make the effort and they often come from the least likely source. Shirley also tells the story of when her son, Jarrett, now nineteen years old, was a high school junior. One young man on his football team was killed by a bullet, fired by a gang member. He was simply on the street at the wrong time. The boy's mother was crushed and in shock for weeks. The high school team decided that the best memorial to their fellow team member was to care for his mother. And care for her they did. They saw that she had a flower on Mother's Day and made sure she was invited to, and attended, team functions. These young athletes, with more than enough friends, school work and activities to fill their time, called her and went by with pizza. That mother was at every home game and even some away games the following year. Needless to say, the team bonded and had a great season. What they did for one family is the thing that Shirley thinks those players will always remember about their senior year. Yes, they were busy, but not too busy to care. Some members of that team still come to see her sons, Gary and Ken, because they are Jarrett's friends, and they know how much a visit means to him.

To me, one of the saddest things about Huntington's Disease is the falling away of people who in the past have said, "I love you." Love is an action. Don't tell me you love me, *show me*.

∽

I Will Fight
BY JEAN ELIZABETH MILLER

Yesterday, Kelly's nurse said something which struck me, at first, as somewhat strange. She said, "Jean, Pat and I both agree that as Kelly's mother you are always looking for things which you feel will benefit Kelly, and we understand that." After a few moments I asked, somewhat irritated, "Are you saying that you both feel that I am reaching out in desperation, looking for things?" She replied, "Oh, no, Jean. We just mean that we can understand your frustration when you find these things, and must wonder why no one else has thought of them."

Later I had dinner with one of my best friends, Janis. We've been friends for thirty-six years and I was telling her about this conversation. Jan said, "You know, Jean, most people faced with a terminal illness eventually get to the point where they accept the disease and let things take their natural path. You don't and never have. Although you've always accepted the fact that Kelly is facing death, you have never, ever, just accepted things just because they "should" be. That is one thing we all admire in you, and don't know where you get the determination to keep fighting for her." I just looked at her and said, "How could you not?"

She went on to say that, "Neither hospice or Kelly's doctors are looking at ways to keep Kelly healthy, because their job is to keep her maintained and in no pain. Yet every time something different happens with Kelly, you research and research until you find a possible solution and are usually right. Most people wouldn't do that." I told her if I didn't do these things, Kelly would have been dead two years ago.

Well, I thought about this all last night. It's because I know that Kelly's support team isn't going to take any extraordinary measures to find out why things are happening to her that I feel compelled to fight these things for her. Maybe my family and friends don't understand because they are not living with death at their door each breathing moment. Maybe the professionals are more concerned with those who have a chance to live, than those that don't. But that doesn't make any of it right.

A person with a terminal illness has as much right to quality care as a person who isn't terminally ill. You can take the empathy. You can get that anywhere. Give me someone who is willing to question every little illness to make sure it's not part of the disease. Give me people who care about the person; the living, breathing, loving person who is at the mercy of everyone else to fight for them. If we are the only ones who can do that for our loved ones, then fight we must. I, for one, could never live with myself again if I didn't.

~

Farewell
BY KIM SIGNORET

There are so many places I wouldn't have gone, so many people I wouldn't have seen and met, so many expeditions I wouldn't have led if I had only known in advance what I was to experience.
—Douchan Gersi

I knew that Albert was at-risk for Huntington's Disease when we chose to have children. In my thoughts, I saw Woody Guthrie. If his mother had known that he would have HD, and then decided not to have children, this world would have missed him. Woody lived such a full life, and he gave us so much... this "pHD" gave us his wonderful music, his son Arlo's music and his wife Majorie's activism.

So this is how Albert and I have lived – we have gone, we have seen, we have met and we have led. Because of this, I now have many, many wonderful memories and two wonderful sons.

Albert was a husband, father, sailor, judo player and engineer. He graduated from the Lycée Franco Mexicano in 1974, and completed a mechanical and industrial engineering degree, with honors, at the Instituto Tecnologico de Estudios Superiores de Monterrey in 1979. He was an alumnus of the University of Wisconsin at Madison, where he earned an M.B.A. in marketing, with honors, in 1983.

On October 8, 1997, Albert decided to stop living with HD. I had such great hopes for an effective treatment for him in the next five years, but he did not share that hope. During the last five years, his life had been closing, though he was not officially diagnosed until April 1996. He fought at each step, but eventually accepted the loss and moved on. During this time, he touched many lives and made many friends. He enjoyed our children and gave all of his time and attention to them.

Our house was not calm. For about two years I lived in a constant state of tension, trying not to upset my husband and make him angry. Our two boys, who are five and ten years old, also felt the tension. An incident in mid-September, when he became overly angry at our five-year-old, set off the final round. My son is still talking about it. Previously, Albert's anger problems had focused on me, but with this incident, and now I've heard about a few others, he was no longer able to control his anger with the kids. At no point was he physically abusive, although I could see that without attention to more medication, we were headed toward some problems.

My husband did not want to be hospitalized, sedated or to have other people making decisions for him. We had arrived at the point where we could no longer work with him directly, but were having to arrange things behind his back. A direct approach enraged him to where he was destructive. My sons and I had to leave the house for three days in mid-September, while he destroyed things in the house. I think he knew that his anger was an issue, although he would not acknowledge it to me or others. I was always the "one in the wrong who caused him to be angry." I "deserved" his anger.

Ultimately, his final days were not spent in anger, but in depression. A car accident in late September was the final straw. He realized that he was not going to be able to continue driving.

There are questions about the drugs he was taking and "what if's." What if I had gotten him to the psychiatrist the day before? What if we had hospitalized him? What if... what if...? I am struggling with these questions and will continue to struggle for some time. I have come to believe that Albert decided a long time ago that he would not live with HD. A childhood friend of his told me that when they were in college, Albert had told him that he would end his life if he had his father's disease.

While I understand his decision, I had such great hopes that new research was going to give us something for him. No matter how bad things were, I was not ready for him to go. And I am angry at him for not waiting longer. But, many people have told me it was his life, his pain, his decision.

I never had the opportunity to tell him goodbye; that is something the children and I will have to live with for the rest of our lives. I hope that my story and my farewell letter to Albert will touch others and in some way help.

Dear Albert,

We miss you. We were not ready for you to leave us. Eric, Alain and I look in every corner of the house and still see you. And when something happens, we talk about what if Daddy were here? He would do this or say that.

But we know that you are at peace. We know you have gone to a place where you are healthy... you can walk without pain and are happy... and we know you are and will be forever with us... You are in the trees, the grass, the flowers, and that bright star we see at night... you are all around us.

We know that your decision to leave us was done with courage, and that you loved us so deeply that you could not bear to be with us, except in love. We understand.

You demanded so much of life and wanted so much. And in the process of living, you experienced so many wonderful things... you were always exploring, you sought adventure and you succeeded at everything you did.

I know, whether you acknowledged it consciously or not, you tried to live up to your grandfather's extraordinary life. And you did! Everything that you loved about his life, you accomplished.

Your spirit was so strong... you had a sense of direction and will power that was so important to us... and you knew how truly important it was to live each day to its fullest.

Eric, Alain and I cherish the example of living that you left us. Rest now in peace and with our love. Farewell, Albert.

Kim

∽

I Really Do Love You, Mom
BY SANDY L.

My mom has Huntington's Disease. She reminds me of the character, Leonard, in the movie, *Awakenings*. She tries so hard to maintain her dignity in various everyday situations. I see people looking at her all the time, and I am sure they're wondering if she's drunk. If my mom was aware of how people perceive her, she'd be mortified. Mom used to pride herself on the fact that she was "classy." She was so classy I still harbor bad feelings about the cotillion and formal manners class that she made me take in junior high.

My mom was very smart; she worked as a bookkeeper for my dad, a self-employed CPA. I remember her as a good, loving mom when I was a child. And she loved to be around people. She had an assertive personality that was at odds with the classy, demure lady she tried to be, and as we got older, she became more pushy and manipulative. This was probably an early symptom of HD, but I guess I thought she was just going through the empty nest syndrome and/or menopause.

My mom is horrible to be with. She denies that anything is wrong with her, and if you bring up the subject of her infirmities, she will change the subject and then jabber on and on. When she does that, I call it her "Eveready Bunny" mode; she just keeps going and going and going.

Sometimes she'll say things that just slug you in the gut; untrue, hurtful stuff about a family member. She sometimes will take a minor grain of truth and blow it out of proportion and then fabricate a tall tale. She has accused people of being sexually abused, going bankrupt, having affairs, and being gay when there is no basis for her comments.

No wonder Mom is lonely. She has alienated friends and family by what she says and does. It is very painful to be with her. I'll see her struggling physically, for example, as we try to walk, and I'll reach out to take her arm. She always yanks it back and then rushes ahead of me. I try to tell her that one can take another person's arm just as a sign of affection, just to walk together, but she can only see it as a sign of frailty.

She is so lonely that she continually wants to party to get the family together. That's all she'll talk about, the next fun event she wants to create or enjoy. But the fun is all in her head because when we get together with her, it's just not fun. We're afraid she'll fall, we can't understand what she is saying due to the slurring of her speech, and quite often it doesn't make sense anyway. We see her struggling to do things like cut meat or get food to her mouth, yet she won't take any help and gets angry at any implication that something is wrong.

My mom is demanding, she doesn't cooperate, and denies she has any problems. My brothers and I don't know what to do with her even after we have tried many ways to help her. We've had meetings with the doctor and minister, gone to look at assisted-living housing, and tried to get her to sign the Power of Attorney forms. She won't take the medication that could go a long way towards helping her live a happier life. As of today, she still lives in the big old brick house that we grew up in. When I try to hire help through the Visiting Nurses Association, she won't allow them in, even though I know living alone is dangerous. We've pleaded with her, shunned her and put up with her. She's just horrible; or rather, the disease has made her horrible.

I have two brothers and, for now, none of us has been tested for the gene. My brothers are avoiding the topic of HD and the inevitable of what will happen to Mom. After a recent trip to the eye doctor regarding Mom's cataract removal, the doctor called me and said that my brothers and I ought to "Put away your own anxieties and sit down and talk about what's best for mom." I agree, but, for some reason, it never happened.

My mom has a strong Christian faith but, because of her degenerating intellect, I know she thinks God is on her side and not ours. Mom is using her faith falsely and that really stirs up the guilt about honoring your parents. Somewhere inside me, I am still her daughter, trying to gain her love, show respect, give her my all. It hurts.

At this writing, my brothers and I have hired an attorney to gain guardianship. Mom is terribly mad and tells me it is "discrimination against senior citizens" and on and on. I did a lot of soul-searching to reach this action. What are my motivations? Somewhere I'm still her teenage daughter who didn't want to be "classy"; am I doing this to get even? Then the forty-year-old me, and the doctor, minister, my brothers, relatives and old family friends remind me that she's a danger to herself, that we are all truly alarmed. No one likes to make hard choices. Sometimes, the best way of showing love means making those tough choices.

∽

Telling the Children...

BY JILL ALAM

Reflections of a conversation between Jill Alam, HD Family Liaison, North and South Carolina, and her seven-year-old daughter.

I, too, have struggled with the issue of telling my children. My husband died of HD and every day I see the devastation of HD. I did not want to tell Adri. She goes with me to a lot of my clients' homes. She sees the disease with children's eyes. She is so kind and loving to my clients. She also recognizes when their condition deteriorates with those child-like eyes.

The issue came to a head one day when she confronted me. She said, "My daddy had HD, right?"

"Yes," I replied.

"Will I have it, Mommy?"

Well, the mommy side of me wanted to scoop her up, lie to her and say, "No, baby, never." The practical side wanted to explain genetics and probabilities. A compromise was quickly reached internally when she said, "Well?"

This was as good a time as any to speak with my baby about the topic I never wanted to speak of. I told her, "You are at-risk for the disease. You may get it, you may not. Either way, I'm here and I will always love you."

In her infinitely wise, seven-year-old way, she said, "If I do get it, I'm glad you're my mommy. You know a lot about it."

∽

Sights and Sounds
BY BRENDA PARRIS SIBLEY

Sometimes it's a sound,
birds like we listened to,
or the music she liked to hear;
Sometimes a smell,
like flowers, or even the
shampoo she used;
Sometimes bacon frying,
or the pudding she liked.
Over and over, every day,
I think of my mother,
and tears flow.
I was so tired, but why
did I give up?
Those were the best times,
the only really important times
in all of my life.

Copyright © 1996, 1997 Brenda Parris Sibley

Brenda's mother suffered from Alzheimer's and her ex-husband currently has Huntington's Disease.

The Bracelet Promise

BY CARMEN LEAL-POCK

The glitter of green stones drew me to the solitary display case. The light bounced off the silver and glass. Amidst the jumble of holiday shoppers, I made my way to the corner area reserved for fine jewelry and gazed upon the bracelet, noticing the unique handiwork. The beaten-silver, fashioned in such a way as to resemble diamond chips, was delightful. Seeing dozens of dark green emeralds, I knew this was a one-of-a-kind treasure.

As I stared in wonder at the intricate piece, I remembered a promise my husband had made. David had bought me a lovely gift four years before on our honeymoon. He had selected an emerald green Austrian crystal and seed pearl bracelet in honor of my May birthstone. As he fastened it on my wrist, he lovingly said, "I promise you that soon I will buy you real emeralds. Just wait." Though I loved the honeymoon gift, deep down I looked forward to David's promise.

Until that time, however, I still delighted in wearing the delicate creation. I wore it frequently, each time remembering the island boutique. Whenever David saw the bracelet, he remembered his promise, and would reassure me that the time was coming soon when he would keep it.

It became our habit over the years to look in every jewelry store window as if searching for the Holy Grail. We wandered in and out of countless shops, becoming discouraged when we realized the cost of the promise was well beyond our means. I soon wavered in my belief that I would ever own what David desired to give me. However, David never lost faith.

Now we were in the mall during the last week before Christmas to buy gifts for our children. Finances were tight; we had agreed there would be no exchange of gifts between us. We had just completed one of the most stressful years possible. With David's diagnosis of Huntington's Disease, our lives had forever changed. This terminal, neurological disorder had pitched us into a panic, not to mention near bankruptcy.

I looked up from the case into David's eyes and saw love shining even brighter than the stones. I could tell in his mind that nothing short of this bracelet would satisfy his honeymoon promise, but I knew there was no way we could possibly afford it. I tried to tell him but the words died on my lips. He'd had so many disappointments this year, I didn't have the heart to tell him the answer was no.

Thinking fast, I came up with a reason to decline what I knew was an offer I could not accept. I have large wrists and normally bracelets don't fit. As the store clerk reverently lifted the object out of the case, I knew it would be too small.

The silver and green made a colorful contrast against my brown skin. I silently acknowledged how much I wanted this bracelet while hoping it would not fit. As the clerk reached around my wrist and closed the intricate clasp, my heart both plummeted and leapt. It fit! It was perfect, yet I knew there was no way we could afford it. The unpaid bills, with more looming in the future, had placed a vise around our checkbook.

I glanced at my best friend and saw his shining smile burst forth. This man, who had never hurt anyone, was now the victim of one of the cruelest diseases known to man. His was a sentence with only one verdict. Death. Untimely, slow and cruel death. My eyes brimmed with tears as I realized we would not live out our dream of growing old together. To David, this was not just one more bauble in an already overcrowded jewelry box. Rather, this was his love displayed on my arm for all the world to see. To David, a promise made was a promise kept. I sadly realized that he might not have many more months or years to keep his promise. Suddenly, it became the most important covenant ever made. Somehow I had to juggle the bills to let him have the honor of keeping his promise.

"Do you like it?" he whispered. Hearing the hope in his voice, mingled with seeing the love in his eyes, was something I am sure few women ever have the privilege of experiencing. It was clear that David cherished me. All he ever wanted, from the day we met, was to please me.

"Yes, honey, I love it." I answered. "It's exactly what I want."

The clerk reached for my arm to remove the bracelet. I could not believe this little object had worked its way into my heart so quickly. "How much is it?" I finally asked. Slowly the man turned over the little white tag. Two hundred fifty dollars, it read. Surely it was a mistake! I had seen enough to know that price was only a fraction of its worth.

The man began to extol the virtues of the item pointing out the one hundred and eighty emeralds in a hand-made Brazilian setting. But even though two hundred fifty dollars was an incredible price, it might as well have been $2,500.00, for all we could stretch our meager budget. Without thinking, I asked, "Would you take two hundred twenty-five dollars, tax included?" I surprised myself at that question because shops in malls do not normally bargain. He looked at me in surprise and answered, "That will be fine."

Before he could change his mind, I whipped out my credit card, all the while watching as David beamed with pride. The man quickly handled the transaction and we were on our way. Every few steps we would stop and look at the bracelet. Before we reached the car, David said, "When I get sicker and eventually die, you need to look at each emerald. Each one will remind you of something special we've done. A trip we took, a movie we saw, or a moment we shared. This will be your memory bracelet." I began to cry. David's concern was not his own failing health, but for how I would handle life without him.

As we worked our way home in the bumper to bumper traffic in rush hour Honolulu, I wondered just how we could pay for the bracelet. Oddly enough, I never really panicked, I was just somehow curious how it would all work out. We talked as we travelled and every so often looked at the miracle of the promise kept.

On the way into the house, I grabbed the mail and began to open it as we walked inside. Amidst the usual bills were two cards. I opened the first which was from a church where I had sung several times that year. It was a thank you note for my music ministry along with a gift. I was speechless. I was looking at a check for two hundred dollars! I reached for the second card and slit it open. Out fell two bills; a twenty and a five. The card was simply signed, "A friend in Christ."

I looked up at David and we both began to laugh. I remembered how I had felt the need to ask the clerk if he would take two hundred twenty-five dollars, tax included. Even as we were in the mall, the payment for David's promise was in the mailbox. God had already taken care of every detail, including the twenty-five dollars plus tax.

It is just a piece of jewelry. Something I could have lived without. But the memories attached to our time together have helped to make me the woman I am today. The exquisite joy and the unspeakable grief of this relationship have grown me in ways I could never have anticipated. The promise David spoke on our honeymoon had been fulfilled. It was only through God that we stopped at that shop on that day to find that specific bracelet. The pastor of a small church, coupled with an unknown friend, listened to God as they decided their holiday giving.

Before I was ever born, God made another promise. He promised me eternal salvation. He promised He would be with me every step of the way. All I had to do was ask. Just as God never stopped believing I would claim that first promise, David never stopped believing in his bracelet promise. When I wear my emeralds, I pull out memories I have tucked away in my heart. I also remember David's faith and God's promises.

∽

Treasured Memories
JEAN ELIZABETH MILLER

Time moves so swiftly and not always forgiving.
I have an abundance of faith in the power of love,
however am forced to acknowledge this faith cannot
spare me from a yet unbearable pain.

Life is so precious and precarious at once.
Treasured memories offer sanctions of tranquility
in a life sometimes filled with uncertainties.

Thank you for being the friend that you are
and one of my most treasured memories.

To My Sister

Anonymous

"Is that our baby? She's smaller than a doll!"
"Well, she came early so she's tiny. Maybe she can wear your doll's clothes..."
I looked at your itty-bitty face and fell in love with you then.
Your pink little nose like a tiny rosebud to me
Wrinkling as you giggled and wriggled and allowed us to fawn
Over you. Tiny you.

You are the third of us. You have been our joy and delight,
Our peacemaker. My friend and at times my only connection to family.
I ran from the raw wounds of HD (how I hate it still today!)
Which meant I ran from you too. And you needed me.
I had to leave in order to grow free from pain and guilt.
Left you. Precious you.

You stayed home and dealt with our sister's decline,
You visited Daddy when nobody else would or could and had to answer,
"Where is she, why doesn't she come?" And you watched him cry.
You told me all this in kindness one day and I swear
My heart ripped with the screech of brakes hit too late.
Daddy was gone. Left you. And me.

So we soldiered on through our sister's last years,
Stood together at Daddy's gravesite that wintry day by the pines.
"How will we remember where he is amidst all this?" you asked.
"From the guard house, go two trees down towards the road.
Two trees that are like you and like me." I hoped then.
Hoped for you and for me.

Our sister, I can't even write her name it hurts me too much,
Died alone without ever getting to share what it felt like in her head.

FACES OF HUNTINGTON'S

What did she think? Did she know we loved her? Did she know we were scared?
Scared for her and for us? Did she know we loved her? She only screamed.
I can't say anymore about her, my heart's ripping again. Hear it screeching?
For you and for me?

You. Always our precious one, the tiniest one. The kindest one.
You loved me always even when I was so sisterly nasty and wretchedly dumb.
Your heart with its congenital "defects" has always been pure and perfect.
You call me now so often. I know you now as a woman. I love you so.
I see you staggering and hear your words slurring. It's ripping again...
For you and for me.

I love you, my sister, with this ripping heart.
Can you hear the song it's singing as it screeches apart?
I love you and want to hold you all the days of your life, however long it is.
I won't let you go without telling you this. My ears are yours to talk to,
I would give you my brain if it would give you a chance.
For you. For you.

To My Child

BY GABRIELLE HAMILTON

To my child
*   to my future*
*   to my love*
*   to my soul*
I write this letter
*   describing how strong*
*   how brave*
*   how smart I was*
in making you
*   so you would know*
*   you would hear*
*   you would feel safe.*

You may sometimes feel cold without me to protect
*   your body*
*   your mind*
*   your spirit*
while I'm held hostage by this hateful disease
*   that has captured the me you wanted to know*
*   but you'll survive because of my efforts*
*   and know that I loved you completely.*

January 24, 1996

5

Lou's Story

BY LOUISE A. WILKINSON

A S a young girl, my grandfather used to scare me when he drove us around. My brothers, sister and I hated the jerky way he drove; one foot on the gas and one on the brake. Often, both were going at the same time, it seemed. He always appeared so nervous and impatient. He just couldn't sit still. Later, it became difficult to understand him when he spoke. Since he had been an alcoholic in his younger years, everyone in the family thought it was nerve damage due to his drinking. My father and uncle (his brother) were also alcoholics, and we wondered if they would turn out the same; bouncing off the walls and flinging their arms around. My father died at age 54 so we never really saw how he turned out. My uncle turned out just the same as Grampa.

We were convinced that alcohol caused it and his doctors all seemed to agree. We, my brothers, sister and I, all knew that we had a predisposition for alcoholism, and each in his own way struggled with it. The only thing, I think, that kept us on track was the fear of turning out the same as Grampa and our uncle. We all joked about them, but secretly feared that we would be the same.

In 1993, two years after my uncle stopped drinking, he was in the hospital because of tuberculosis that he has in five separate locations throughout his body. While in the hospital, a doctor saw him and she recognized Huntington's symptoms. Although that word was mentioned about Grampa, I don't think he was ever tested as there was no DNA testing available. No one really took it seriously because we didn't know enough about it. Again, we attributed his symptoms to alcohol.

My uncle was tested and told that he had Huntington's disease. At first, we all felt bad for him. But we didn't know enough about the disease to be concerned. We talked to my aunt about it. My cousin, their daughter, sent me some abstracts about the disease from medical journals. After reading them, I started to think about the possibilities that it was genetic and that I could have it.

For years, since my mid-thirties, I had been feeling that something wasn't quite right about me. I couldn't put my finger on it, but other people in the family would say things like, "You're just like your uncle, clumsy and forgetful." I was consistently getting worse. I never slept well at night. I seemed to have the need to move all the time. My legs were never still. I also noticed when I was teaching, my speech didn't come as easily anymore and my mind would go blank for one or two seconds. I was having more and more trouble remembering students' names – even students that were very familiar to me.

Although everyone experiences these things, in the back of my mind, I knew that the occurrences were too frequent to ignore. I began developing coping mechanisms and excuses for tripping, falling down and for my stumbling speech. I would say I had too much on my mind, or I was tired, which was also true. I seemed to second-guess myself all the time and went over things many times so that I wouldn't forget appointments or meetings. I even frequently forgot to check my day book. My school schedule was difficult to keep straight as there were always so many things going on at the same time. I often got confused. I still do, but I manage.

When I learned about the Huntington's, inside, I knew. Everyone else said that I was worrying too much and making it worse; everyone, that is, except my husband and my kids. My husband had been concerned about me and knew that it wasn't "normal" forgetfulness or clumsiness.

It took me several months to decide to get tested. I guess I've always been one to want to know for sure about things because my mind drives me crazy wondering. I obsess. My husband and I talked for hours about it. We talked to my aunt about her life with my uncle. She said that she may have been far less frustrated and judgmental had she known his behavior wasn't just because of his drinking. My uncle had severe mood swings and was miserable and nasty much of the time. He had no patience with anyone, especially with anyone telling him he had no patience. He had bad moods and got frustrated easily. I related to that as well. I had even been put on anti-depressants and had to get therapy for rage attacks in my late thirties. My aunt said that my uncle showed those symptoms in his thirties.

What really convinced me to get tested was my uncle. By the time my uncle retired from work, he was too far into the disease to do all the things they had planned. He can't golf much anymore and their plans to go to Arizona every winter have become very hard on them. My aunt has to do most if not all the driving. He is only sixty-seven years old and he has trouble eating in restaurants as he can't sit still and chokes often. He is always falling or banging into things. In the last year, he has broken ribs and a wrist, as well as sporting several bruises on his body all the time. This also happens to me except I don't break things because I am more careful than he is. At first, many people thought he was drunk when he went to a restaurant. Since they live in a small town, everyone is getting used to him now.

We decided if I had the disease we would plan our lives for an earlier retirement and move to a better climate without the ice and snow. Also, we decided that a small town would be better as my uncle has lots of support where he is. I contacted the genetics department at the Children's Hospital and went in for a consultation. I was shown a video on Huntington's but it was mostly about the team that would be working with me: a counselor, a psychiatrist and a neurologist. Each of them spoke but none of them really explained what to expect. It seemed that I wasn't much more informed about the disease, but maybe that was because it never sank in at the time. I did much research on my own. The counselor and the psychiatrist saw me a couple of times, and I only met the neurologist once. For the most part, they seemed to be interested in finding out whether I could handle the results, positive or negative. I was frustrated with having to wait. I just wanted to get on with it.

In my heart, I already knew, and I guess I was looking for validation. It angered me when I talked about my symptoms and all I heard was, "Well, everyone experiences those things. That doesn't mean it's Huntington's symptoms." That phrase drove me to distraction, I heard it so many times. I thought, "Do they think I'm stupid? I know everyone does these things. That's one of the reasons Huntington's goes undiagnosed for so long." There was always some "explanation" for these things. But, I know me. I've lived in this body with this mind for forty-five years and watched two people with Huntington's in my family. I knew.

I did understand friends and family downplaying it, but not the "experts." The one exception was the psychiatrist who said that everyone knows their own bodies and minds better than everyone else. "Thank you," I thought. The rest don't matter because it's irrelevant whether anyone else thinks it's Huntington's or not. I have to live with it and compensate, whether it's psychosomatic or not.

After about three months, I had an appointment with the genetic counselor and the neurologist to get the results. My husband went with me, and I have to admit I was nervous. When we got the results and they were positive, I had mixed feelings. The neurologist kept saying that I had the gene but that didn't necessarily mean that I was showing symptoms. That's like being a little pregnant. She kept saying that I wasn't showing any neurological symptoms and as far as she was concerned, I didn't have the disease yet. Now this was based on pricking my feet and watching me walk. I had been telling her about my symptoms all along, and there she was telling me that I didn't have any.

I remember a nurse once telling me after eighteen hours of labor that the pains and contractions could stop at any time and I would be sent home because I hadn't dilated yet. That was the worst feeling in the world. Excuse me, that baby was coming whether I looked like it or not! I felt the same this time. I just wanted to get out of that office as fast as I could. Talk about an emotional reaction. But at least inside I finally had my validation and knew that I wasn't crazy. It didn't really matter what name the doctors put on it. I had wondered for years what was going on with my mind, and now I knew.

For the first few weeks after finding out, I intellectualized everything. I went about accepting the news on the level of practicality. What do we do now? I talked about it to my family and a few friends. Most of them had the same reaction we initially had. What is Huntington's? What does it do to you? Is it contagious? Don't worry about it, I do those things too, everyone does.

Over the next six months, everything I did and said, I related to the disease. I got depressed watching my uncle and read everything that I could get my hands on. I obsessed. At first, I was afraid to tell my colleagues. I told most of them, one by one, as an opportunity arose. At times I even used it as an excuse, letting my mistakes be explained away. I revisited the psychiatrist on a few occasions. He kept reassuring me that I was going through a normal response. I guess the things that scared me the most were the thoughts of dementia and helplessness. I'm an artist, and the thought of not having control over my muscles is terrifying to me.

My older brother went into total denial at first. He just didn't want to think about it. I didn't press him and since we weren't close anyway, he was able to put it off for several months. My sister worried a little more, but didn't want to get tested as she was getting married again, has no children and is financially secure. She doesn't think it would make much of a difference anyway and feels that she doesn't have any of the symptoms.

My brother called one day and asked me why I got tested. In the beginning, I thought it was only my choice to be tested. Then I realized the results would affect my husband and sons. I told my brother I got tested for my husband and children because of what my aunt went through, having to live with it. I felt my husband deserved the right to prepare himself for the future.

I mentioned that his wife and their five children had a right to plan their lives. A couple of months later, my brother decided to get tested. He is presently going through the prediagnostic period and we haven't talked about it.

Our youngest brother would like to get tested, but lives so far from any major city that it isn't feasible for him to do it at this time. He is about 19 hours from Vancouver, which is the nearest genetic testing center. I know he and his wife worry about it though.

My friends reacted in several different ways. Our best friends arrived with a teddy bear mom hugging a baby to help me feel better. They have been very supportive. We joke about it with them and are able to be completely natural with each other. Other friends backed off. Still others, more casual acquaintances, don't treat me any differently. Some treated me like an invalid at first.

Professionally, I reacted very strongly. At first I felt a great loss because I was ambitious and was heading for administration in the Arts Council. I was on several committees and had plans. My immediate reaction was to quit my committee work as I couldn't keep my mind on it and felt that there was no use anyway. I also decided not to pursue a high school teaching position, opting for a safe environment until long term disability kicked in. I was scared.

Time passes even with Huntington's Disease, and somehow I have managed to get through each day. I realized how much I love teaching and so I now have a high school position and I'm planning to go back to my committee work. I have even joined a theater group and am going to be doing dinner theater. I will admit that, although my fears have settled down, they will always be there, and I know that I have to live my life to its fullest.

My husband and I are not as complacent as we used to be. We are trying to enjoy life as it comes and are consciously not putting things off. We bought the house we were renting and more life insurance. We have set definite goals for the future. We play a lot of golf and I have really taken an interest in my garden. We put in a goldfish pond and fountain in the back yard and find it is a great place to relax when things get us down. I'll also admit that Huntington's Disease is still on my mind. However, it is not ruling my thoughts, and I have settled down quite a bit. Life goes on.

I think the prediagnostic testing is helpful, but feel that three months is too long to wait. Most people have been waiting and wondering for a time before they decide to get tested. I think more information should be available and patients' fears should never be downplayed. They are real. I also feel that a person should wait until they have to make some life decisions before getting tested. It may be difficult, if not impossible, to get insurance once the diagnosis is done. I am very glad that I had my children before I got tested because it may have influenced whether or not I had children. I feel that since the disease does not manifest itself until the children are almost adults, in my case anyway, it would have been a shame not to have had my boys. They are handling it well and are very supportive.

It is also possible that I may not have gone back to University and gotten a degree at the age of thirty-seven had I known about having Huntington's Disease. I would not be a teacher now. I have been very happy teaching and have made a difference to many students.

Because there are so many considerations before going through with testing, I think the prediagnostic counseling should be thorough. What are the symptoms? What is the worst case scenario? What should a person think about before getting tested? These are some of the things that candidates for testing should know.

The end of the school year is only weeks away and this has been quite a year for me. I guess because I started the new job and am no longer in my comfort zone, I have been hyper-sensitive to the disease. I also took on the acting and found it stressful, but fun. It's almost as if I have to fit an entire lifetime into a short period of time.

My symptoms have definitely increased. I notice a big difference between the beginning of the year and now. This year has been tough as the myoclonus* seizures are bad – over one hundred a day if I don't take my medication. Even with the medication, I still jerk when I'm relaxed. It is not that difficult to swallow but I am now conscious of it because sometimes it takes me two or three tries before I get something down. I almost never eat anything without a liquid. It seems as if there is always a dry spot about two inches down my throat. I also have to clear my throat a lot.

I have "come out of the closet," so to speak, at work with the administration. I am very fortunate to have security in my job and realize that it must be terrifying for others who do not. I am free to talk about the disease now, though I spent my first year at this school trying to keep it from the principal and vice-principals. I wanted them to see me as a normal teacher. It worked. They didn't know and said that I would always have a job teaching there if I was able and not to worry, they would be supportive.

Another year passed by, where did it go? It seems as if time is more precious now than ever and when I lose my

---

* Myoclonus is an irregular involuntary contraction of a muscle.

sense of time, I am sad. This has been an eventful year. My youngest son has now graduated and both are working full time, so they are in and out of the house a lot. They have a core group of about nine friends that all hang out together and our house is the central meeting place. Since they're both of age, the beer usually comes here too.

I find that I can't tolerate it as I used to, and they have to walk behind my chair from the back door, through the family room, and downstairs to the fourth level, "the dungeon," I call it. The constant traffic irritates me and makes me nervous. When I'm watching television, I tend to get lost now, and they will come up behind me and give me a hug or kiss and say, "Hi, Mom." At 11:00 p.m. and later, it's a bother so we've had to put a stop to it. It's a small thing that never used to phase me at all; now it does.

Roy, my wonderful husband, is on twenty-four hour alert now and I feel sorry for him. He always was a caregiver, but now I know he has to check everything for me. I forget to turn things off or I start something and then get distracted two or three times. Sometimes I forget what I was doing in the first place. I'll be looking for something, I seem always to be looking for something I misplaced, and I'll see something that I haven't seen for a while. That will start me off on a new journey. I am sure it's as frustrating for Roy as it is for me.

I have several things that I have started and never finish; ironing is my worst. Roy asked me two weeks ago to shorten some shorts for him but there they sit. I bought two sheets to sew together to make a cover for our futon, but there they sit. I still haven't painted my two cement frogs that were blasted in the last hail storm, but there they sit. I just can't seem to follow through with tasks and then I forget all about them until the next time. When I think of it, most of the time I don't have the energy or motivation to do anything.

As wonderful as the administration has been, it is getting more difficult to do my job each day. My memory is getting more erratic and I have trouble typing. I have been trying to make a decision this summer about whether to keep teaching. My neurologist, psychiatrist and physician all think that I should quit, as it is too draining and taking all of my energy. I have to agree. I don't have to worry about money as I have long term disability insurance through my job and a pension that I can get from the government. Once I am not working, it will be like getting a raise. I am unsure about giving up such an important part of my life. I love teaching and teaching loves me. The problem isn't the teaching so much as the planning, scheduling and marking. Sometimes the kids wait two weeks to get projects marked, and believe me, in high school they let you know.

So I have pretty well decided not to go back this fall. It will be better for the school if I don't go back in September. This way, they will be able to hire a teacher for the entire year, instead of a replacement in December.

Loretta, my HD social worker, has lots for me to do for the HD community. I think it may just give me the grounding and focus that I'll need while I adjust to being a lady of leisure. I don't want to feel as if I'm useless and I don't want my brain to go into neutral, watching soap operas all the time and forgetting to wash my hair. I belong to a spa, so now I'll have time and energy to get there regularly since it's going to be part of my routine. I intend to become more involved with our local Huntington's chapter and do other types of volunteering as long as possible. Just because I am slowing down with HD, it doesn't mean I am not still the same gregarious person who embraces life. I still need people in my life and have a lot to give to those in need.

My sons, who are still living at home, will be company for me, and I have Duffy, my toy poodle, who follows my every step. I have to admit that it is pretty hard for Duffy with the chorea. The hardest part is going to be my poor husband coming home tired, and I'll be ready to do something. He's a real homebody and doesn't like going out much. It's been a problem for years and I fear that the more dependent I become, the more house bound I'm going to be.

Yesterday was a big news day. They have discovered that over time, protein forms clumps on the brain cells of individuals who have the gene for HD. The clumps eventually trigger the death of those cells. This is such good news for everyone who has HD, and those at-risk. I am glad they are so close now because there is hope for my sons as well as for me.

∽ 6

Faces of Humor

BY CARMEN LEAL-POCK

I know God will never give me more than I can handle, I just wish He didn't trust me so much.

—Mother Teresa

Humor is a balm to the soul. We all need it if we're to make it through life, because on the roads which we all travel, there are bumps, and smooth spots, and sharp curves, and potholes. It's just that some roads are bumpier that others. During the hard times, memories of the good times somehow makes the bumps a little smoother. Let me tell you something funny that happened to me before I had even heard of Huntington's Disease.

Before Huntington's entered my life, like everyone else, I had "phases" of my life when nothing seemed to go right. Sometimes they were relatively short; one or two days maybe. Sometimes, things didn't straighten out for longer periods; weeks, months, or even years when life seemed just a series of hardships.

Some years back, that was the story of my life. My first marriage was a battle zone; I worked at a stressful, high powered, corporate America job, and had two very young children I was doing my best to raise. On top of that, my boss was a Class-A jerk. Each day was like living a nightmare. Although I have always been an optimistic person, at that time I found little humor in living; I could not shake the panic that crept into my heart each morning.

Sometimes, if we're dealt a particularly bad hand in life, we inherit a boss like the one I found myself stuck with. His name was Mr. You Produce And I'll Take All The Credit. But to give him his due, he did do one thing well; he was great at delegating. Easy system; I did everything, he did nothing.

One morning, I was filling in for him once again. I had to give a major presentation to a group of high-level, crème de la crème potential customers. This was an important discourse, expected to whet their commercial appetites for our product. But this wasn't supposed to be my talk, and I was angry. No, I was not in what could be construed as a happy sales mood. That was the day of my son's Christmas program, and I was supposed to be there. Instead, there I was having to give the "dog and pony show" again. To make matters worse, the luncheon was at a hotel attached to the largest mall in Hawaii. Parking was at a premium and traffic was what you would expect a week before Christmas.

At the time, our new cellular phone company was in its infancy, and there were less than twelve units up and running. One perk of being a manager was that I had a phone and used it often. Service was not going to be open to the public until June. Back then, I used a car phone versus a portable.

That day, I parked the car and continued talking on my car phone. That meant keeping the keys in the ignition.

After I'd completed my conversation, I hung up and got out. Naturally, the split second I shut the door I realized that I'd locked myself out of the car. My literature, business cards, and everything else I needed for my speech were tantalizingly there... within sight but out of reach, in the locked car. I was in a panic!

Then I remembered the unlocked hatchback. Great! All I had to do was to crawl over the seat, get the keys and go get this lousy thing over with.

Now, I'm sure everyone knows that Hawaii is a casual place. However, for this very important talk, I was in full, big city business regalia. I even had on shoes and pantyhose. And as I did not want a panty line showing through the tight straight skirt, I did what other women do whether they admit it or not; I went without underwear.

I'm sure by now your imaginations are running rampant, and you can see where this is going. As I shimmied into the car and over the seats, my dress rode up around my waist and though I honestly tried to pull it down as I went, I couldn't use too much force because I was afraid of ripping it. Just a little more and I'd make it!

"I don't know whether to arrest you for breaking and entering or indecent exposure."

A young police officer, trying to contain his laughter, asked me to step out of the car.

Looking past him, I saw a little crowd had formed. Somehow, I managed to extricate myself, after which I rapidly pulled my dress down.

"You see officer," I began, "I was in my car, talking on the phone...."

Cellular phones were not commonplace back then, and it was evident he didn't believe me. It took some time to persuade the officer to unlock the doors and let me prove my case. All the while the crowd was growing as people told and retold the story of my embarrassing moment. Once I'd convinced him that I wasn't some sort of exhibitionist, I retrieved the car phone and showed it to the policeman and the gathered crowd. Smiling gallantly at the many jokes that were being tossed around, I passed out business cards galore.

The police officer didn't write me a ticket and everyone had a great laugh at my expense. Everyone, that is, except me. Things were definitely not going my way. I was missing my son's program, had been placed in a very embarrassing situation, was almost late for the presentation, and my dress was wrinkled.

If I could just get through this I was going to quit. But I was going to tell my boss off first, then I was going to quit. Imagine my surprise when I marched into the room and received a standing ovation. It seems a large part of the primarily male group had caught my act in the parking lot. Talk about an ice breaker.

I had a choice; I could walk away in humiliated indignation, or do the talk without a shred of humor. But there was a third choice, too. I figured I was probably going to laugh about it someday, and I might as well laugh about it then. Taking a deep, sweeping bow, I laughed. The atmosphere in the room turned it into a party. For a time, I had no worries at all and I was having fun. I hadn't laughed in such a long time. It felt great. You know what else? It turned out to be one of the best sales presentations I ever did and I ultimately sold many phones later that year to people who had first viewed the phone while viewing me.

Now, sometimes when I reach a real rough spot in the road of life that I'm traveling, I remember this and laugh. Because it was funny then, and it's still funny now. And I need to laugh as much now as I did then. In fact, I need it more.

I know that living with Huntington's Disease is far worse than any of my embarrassing moments. I truly cannot think of a more insidious, unlaughable disease. But there are funny things that do happen in the course of living with HD just as there are in every other course of life.

I have a friend from the on-line support group who has two adult sons with HD. Shirley has a great sense of humor as she tells the story of her two sons who live in a little trailer in the back of the main house. Their separate living quarters helps them maintain their dignity and independence. As her sons have a penchant towards sweets and overeat if they are left around, Shirley tried to make the trailer safe and free of anything that would be harmful if eaten. But Shirley's sister was moving and had temporarily placed some bags containing odds and ends in the refrigerator. One day, Shirley walked in and saw her sons looking like the cats who had swallowed the canary. One had a piece of foil almost to his mouth, and there was a little box of Preparation H sitting between them. She had caught them just in time. They thought it was candy. All three laughed and laughed when the boys found out what it was. They decided that laughter was a better medicine than Preparation H.

Shirley's oldest son calls Huntington's Disease the M & M disease. He says that it sure messed up his mind and muscles, and it's not even a piece of cake or candy.

Even though some days it doesn't feel like it, there is life beyond HD. We still have jobs and families and activities that can all afford us some humor. It is all around us. All we have to do is be observant.

Most of these actual signs, found somewhere in America, come under the "Duh!" category, but they made me chuckle. Keep your eyes peeled for humor everywhere.

In a Los Angeles dance hall: Good cle
night but Sunday.

On a Maine shop: Our motto is to give o
the lowest possible prices and workmansh

On a display of "I love you only" valentine cards: Now available in multi-packs.

In the window of a Kentucky appliance store: Don't kill your wife. Let our washing machine do the dirty work.

In a clothing store: Wonderful bargains for men with sixteen and seventeen necks.

Outside a country shop: We buy junk and sell antiques.

In the window of an Oregon store: Why go elsewhere and be cheated when you can come here?

My favorite part of the Tonight Show is when Jay Leno reads off newspaper headlines submitted by his viewers. Here are a few that have come across my desk.

Police begin campaign to run down jaywalkers.
Two convicts evade noose, jury hung.
Miners refuse to work after death.
Two Soviet ships collide – one dies.
If strike isn't settled quickly it may last a while.
War dims hope for peace.
Smokers are productive, but death cuts efficiency.
Cold wave linked to temperatures.
Child's death ruins couple's holiday.
Something went wrong in jet crash, experts say.

Lack of water hurts ice fishing.
Yellow snow tested for nutrition.

Despite the positive effects of humor, there are some people who think laughter is useless. The comic strip is never to be read and all movies viewed must be dramas. Disease is a serious thing. Laughter is nothing more than a waste of time. If that is the way they feel, no wonder their lives are so hard

Life is a continual series of opportunities sprinkled with crisis. I know of no one who has opportunities without difficulties. When we can live our lives with dignity and hope and humor, the difficulties are more easily managed and there is more joy.

Laughter is as essential to our well-being as food and water. It is an emotional release that allows us to continue to function in stressful situations. A hearty laugh speeds up the heart rate, improves blood circulation and works muscles all over the body. Laughter eases tension, stress and anger. We know that depression makes us all susceptible to disease. And, while we also know there is a lot to be depressed about with HD, laughter can help relieve depression. Researchers of the brain have long agreed that laughter activates the release of endorphins, the body's own pain-reducing substance. Without humor, life can be filled with physical pain as well as being grim. Laughter may not cure it, but it helps all of us fight the effects of HD.

During that phase of my life when everything was going wrong, I should have laughed more. Like so many lessons, we know what we should do and we don't do it. Instead of continuing to laugh, I let the weight of my world crush me and I stopped laughing. I also got pneumonia and temporary asthma. I had such a severe attack I almost died.

Watching my dear husband suffering with Huntington's is infinitely worse than going through my divorce. My divorce nearly cost me my sanity and twenty thousand dollars; this is costing me someone I love, my home, my business, countless dollars and so much more. Except for an earache, I have not been sick one day since Dave was diagnosed. One of the differences this time around is laughter. I am making a conscience effort to laugh. I am well and I believe laughter will help me stay that way.

There is so little we can control about Huntington's. There is no cure and we can't control the steady progression of destruction, nor the pace it takes. We can't control who of our beloved families will end up with the gene and become symptomatic. We can't control other people and the way they react to the news. We often feel so helpless over something so seemingly powerful as Huntington's. Laughter, however silly or short lived, gives us power and control. We feel carefree and hopeful during periods of laughter.

Mark Twain said, "The human race has only one really effective weapon, and that's laughter. The moment it arises, all our hardnesses yield, all our irritations and resentments slip away, and a sunny spirit takes their place."

Marsha wrote to me about her two step-children who are at-risk for Huntington's. Their mother is 38 years old and in a nursing home in the final stages. Last year she took the mother and the kids to a support group meeting. As they were sitting there, the thirteen-year-old leaned over and said to Marsha, "Mom, I think I have HD."

She whispered back to him, "Andrew, why do you think you have HD?"

"Everyone here that has HD is wearing glasses and I wear glasses."

She smiled at him, trying to keep from laughing out loud and said to him, "Andrew, look at me. Do I wear glasses?" He answered yes and she asked, "Do I have HD?" "No," he answered.

She placed her arm around him and said, "Don't sweat the small stuff!" He looked at her and smiled the biggest smile she'd seen on him in a long time! They had a great laugh and it helped.

Such a burden to be thirteen and see your mother in a nursing home and have the knowledge that you could have that same disease. Of course he felt powerless and fearful. Of course he was looking for signs. Marsha was so right. Don't sweat the small stuff and take the time to laugh.

I have to remember that I cannot dictate most situations that happen to or around me. I am especially touched when a person with HD is able to keep laughing. At a support group meeting, a woman shared that her husband with HD had fallen one day. She asked him what he was doing down there. He responded by saying the Governor had promoted him to carpet inspector, and he was just trying to get a better look at their carpet. This man has very little control over his muscles and his ability to stay upright is gone. Where others might have found the fall humiliating and been filled with a sense of hopelessness, he was able to laugh. At that moment, I bet he didn't feel powerless at all.

Another man shared that his wife told him they are going to bring children to see her in the nursing home. The children will be told, "This is what will happen to you if you don't eat your vegetables." I think her humor has made it easier for both of them.

There are days when I am cutting through the red tape of medical programs and nothing seems humorous. When

Dave is severely paranoid and we can't seem to adjust his medication to the correct dosage, I have to really work hard at finding humor.

None of us enjoys going to the doctor. Poor Shirley has not one but two affected sons. She plans their appointments together so she doesn't miss more time from work. While I can sympathize with Shirley and her plight, I had to laugh as she outlined a typical day at the doctor's office. Her son Ken usually feels that he needs exercise and has to be chased up and down the halls. He becomes quite agitated if you catch him and she becomes agitated if she doesn't. Then the doctor runs in and out tending to four cases at once and almost forgets who they are and again tries to give them more Haldol. The doctor gets disturbed because she married a man with HD and had three at-risk kids even though she has told him she didn't know he had HD. Next, they leave and the elevator is often not functioning. Once a man's leg was hanging out as the door tried to shut. She and her guys have to take the stairs. Remember, both of her adult sons have chorea. I shudder at the picture of their downward descent. She almost pulls their belt loops off the pants trying to hold on so they don't fall. The van is usually parked two blocks away and they fight to get across the busiest street in Shreveport. By the time they are home from the four-hour junket, she is so glad they have a prescription for Zoloft. Forget the boys, she says, she needs it herself.

I make it a point to start my day with humor. Because I am on the computer so much, I open my day with laughter. I subscribe to humor lists. When I open my morning E-mail, there are jokes to make me laugh. My Internet opening page is the comic strips. I can read a wide range of funnies to make me laugh. The advantage of this is I don't have to read the gloom of the daily news to get to the funnies. I keep a humor file in my computer and have even added a humor link to my web page.

We all need humor in our lives to get us through, no matter what our lives consist of. We are all unique and find humor in different ways. Many things can be done to find humor.

- Surround ourselves with positive people
- Find and tell jokes
- Go to the Comedy Club
- Watch funny movies, cartoons, and television shows
- Look for funny signs and newspaper headlines
- Look for humor in every day situations.
- Subscribe to magazines like Reader's Digest and read every joke or funny story
- Laugh at Country Western song titles

Here are some titles I love. Now I ask you, how can you fail to see the humor in these real songs?

"Her Teeth Were Stained, But Her Heart Was Pure"
"I Don't Know Whether to Kill Myself or Go Bowling"
"I Fell in a Pile of You and Got Love All Over Me"
"I Flushed You From the Toilets of My Heart"
"I Would Have Wrote You a Letter, But I Couldn't Spell Yuck!"
"If My Nose Were Full of Nickels, I'd Blow It All On You"
"If You Don't Leave Me Alone, I'll Go and Find Someone Else Who Will"
"You Were Only a Splinter As I Slid Down the Bannister of Life"
"You're the Reason Our Kids Are So Ugly"

Ecclesiastes 3:4 tells us there is "a time to weep and a time to laugh, a time to mourn and a time to dance." There are times when we all have to grieve and work through our losses with tears. That is natural. Humor does have a very real place in our lives. Laughter is a powerful, positive medicine. The nice thing about humor is, it's accessible to anyone. And it's free. Or at least it's a real bargain.

One day, I was wading through a stack of bills trying to decide which ones to pay and what to do with the rest. The Reader's Digest renewal form fluttered to the table. Without hesitation, I wrote a check for $17.45. I consider that therapy. Each month I open the pages of the magazine and find stories that make me cry. Shedding tears for people I have never met is somehow easier than crying for myself and Dave. Just when I feel wrung dry, I turn the page and find myself laughing hysterically. The difficulties in my life disappear for a few minutes. Whether I plow through the magazine in one sitting or savor a little each day, the laughter and tears help bring peace and joy to my soul.

Yes, Huntington's Disease is hard and we all suffer in varying degrees regardless of whether we have HD, or are at-risk, or are a caregiver. Suffering, however, is not surrendering, and we don't have to let life or HD defeat us.

Laughter

BY GABRIELLE HAMILTON

I'm still laughing
though there are
tears in my eyes
and on my face.
Though my smile may appear
forced and unconvincing.

I'm still laughing
though sometimes
living hurts just as much as dying.
Though being strong
makes me feel weak.

I'm still laughing
though I'm preoccupied
and anxious about the future.
Though there is nothing
I can do
to make things different.

I'm still laughing
because if I stopped
I would become someone else
that I've never met before
and I might not even like.

August 11, 1995

∽7

Christopher's Story

BY CHRISTOPHER CLINE (LEGAL ADOPTED NAME)
R.W. HAVENS (BIRTH NAME)

I SIT alone, wondering if the marauding army lies in wait to attack the strength of my body and the power and creativity of my mind. But, what I am realizing every day now since I learned of this disease is that I am not alone. Some 30,000 people are affected and challenged by this terminal neurological assault. And I sit alone, now wondering if I am the next victim. I didn't really know I could carry this gene and be at-risk. It was a surprise and a shock when I found out that I could be dealing with a fifty percent risk factor, but it really didn't bother me. I guess because I have spent the majority of my life working with, caring for, and being around all kinds of disease.

I was born in Charleston, South Carolina, at the Medical Hospital where most unwed mothers go to deliver. My mom had just finished basic training at Parris Island, and had received her exit physical when she was notified. Her pregnancy was a surprise since her entrance physical had not shown her carrying me, and she had gone through two and a half months of basic training. I now know why the first part of my trip was so bumpy. Eventually, Mom went to live at a local home for girls who were sharing this situation. I never really took the time to try to understand why Mom decided to leave me there in Charleston. But now, after all these years, I realize she was doing what she could; she really didn't have a choice and I now know she wanted me to have a chance. Some thirty years went by between the day I showed up, and the day I got the phone call.

There was really nothing special about July 24, 1996. It was your typical summer day in South Carolina, with the humidity up to eighty percent and the air conditioner pumping away. I was busy going through many papers in the big notebook. The big notebook contained over twenty-five years of names, addresses, phone numbers, facts, hearsay, and recorded stories of who I was and where I came from. I had been searching on and off since I was old enough to understand that a person could have two mothers at the same time.

My adopted mother was extremely helpful, especially after Dad's breast cancer took him from us. She was even more excited about it than I was, but I had this inner need, this primal instinct to find my birth mom after all this time. I had genuinely tried over the years, but to no avail. I felt a sense of satisfaction that I had, however, reunited over two hundred people in those few short years. But for me, my search continued. I poured over all the information in the big notebook and as I reached a page I hadn't been to in a while, something jumped out at me. Something my caseworker had said several years back.

I took the information and called my friend, Marie, and asked her if she could do anything with it. Marie was a wonderful soul, a woman of great love, strength, and courage when it came to adoption. She immediately recognized the information and told me she would get back to me. I sat there for a few minutes and I thought about what I had done with the big notebook all these years. Now Marie and I were going to add yet another page of information. This began to color my already lonely world a little bluer and I shut the notebook and put it back on the shelf.

I sat there and thought to myself, "Well, tomorrow will mark yet another birthday and I will again battle demons of all kinds. Too much alcohol, too much chocolate, too much food, too much of everything, but I guess once a year isn't too bad. I wonder if she will think about me tomorrow, if she will remember that she brought me into this world and left me to fend for myself." And then I thought, "No, she wouldn't just leave me, she was leaving a gift for someone else who could not have their own." And sure enough, we were all blessed.

I continued my day, making phone calls, writing more on my novel, talking to Mother (the one here) and listening to some good music. Before I realized it, the day had turned to evening, and I finally felt the exhaustion from the heat and the emotional roller coaster I had ridden all day. I turned to the pile of pillows and crawled in and amongst them for solace and comfort.

The next morning I awoke to that disgusting sound of the phone ringing before the alarm, and, because it was my special day, I remained amongst the pillows and listened for the machine. I heard Marie's voice singing "Happy Birthday" with a special level of excitement in her voice, and I sat straight up in bed. As I listened to her last note, I realized what I was about to hear. As I sprang from the bed, falling over everything on the floor, I heard Marie say through her laughter and tears, "Chris, we have a match! Call me."

As I reached the phone, she hung up. I stood there holding the phone and listening to the recorded message of the operator, "If you would like to make a call...." I stood there transfixed by my image in the mirror at the end of the hall as the sun beamed across my chest. A breeze blew in through the bathroom window and my skin tightened as the cool air blew across my body. I stood there as the tears began to flow and I watched myself in the mirror, thanking God for my re-birthday present. As I began to regain my senses, I went straight to the coffee pot and started my daily ritual. This was followed by my shower and the realization that I had a phone call to make.

When Marie answered, I could hear the excitement in her voice, and I felt our long search was nearing completion. She gave me all the information and as she told me what she knew, my anxiety and heartbeat increased tenfold. I realized I was only a phone call away from speaking to my birth mother, or so I thought.

The problem was that we had names but no addresses or phone numbers. We only had the name of her hometown. So I took the information and decided no matter what the cost, I was going to call as many of the public libraries as possible in that particular part of the country. I would speak with anyone I could. I had three numbers; someone at one of them had to be able to tell me something. After an hour or so on the phone with someone at the state library, I ended up finding out it would take four to six weeks before the information I had requested could even be verified and sent to me by registered mail. My heart began to plummet as it always had when hitting a dead end, but this time I was not going to accept "no" for an answer. I immediately dialed the county library and received the same basic information and was informed that it would be closing in the next hour. I thanked the librarian and hung up, my heart and hopes dropping to the floor even farther, but I was determined not to stop.

As I looked up through my tears, I realized there was one number left, the city library in my birth mother's hometown. I called immediately, and as it was ringing, I said, "Lord, put an angel on the other end of this line." The sweetest little voice answered. I spoke with the lady for a few minutes asking for the special books I was looking for.

The angelic voice on the other end said sweetly, "Honey, what exactly are you looking for? I don't need those books, I was here then." I told her the address and she immediately replied, "Hon, that's the old Haven's House and one of the girls still lives there." My heart stopped for several beats. I had found my aunt. We continued to talk and she inadvertently mentioned my aunt's husband's name. As she was about to hang up, she said, "Honey, I know this is important, and I am sure she wouldn't be mad. I think she needs to talk to you so let me get the number."

Again my heart stopped a few beats and as she read the number off to me, tears began to form. "She might be home, go ahead and give her a call. And dear, God bless you." I thanked her and as I hung up, I sat speechless and could not move. The tears flowed as I sat there and thought about all the years of dead end searches and all the reunions I had witnessed. Finally, it was my turn.

As I composed myself, I realized I had the phone and was dialing my friend. She answered and all I could say was, "Marie, I found her!" She screamed with such force I thought she was having a coronary. She demanded that I come over and I did, my aunt's number in hand.

When I arrived, Marie and I sat and talked about many things. Then I asked her if she would call and talk with my aunt to verify that we had indeed found my birth mother's beginnings. She collected herself and dialed. Aunt Di answered the phone and Marie began asking all kinds of questions after initially introducing herself. Aunt Di was very informative. All of a sudden, I noticed Marie's expression change and I felt my throat knot. I knew what I was about to hear when Marie said, "Oh, she's in California now?" She looked at me but with a tempered excitement and I froze. She finished the conversation, said "thank you" and hung up.

I never expected Marie to tell me what was to follow. After all the years of searching, I had put myself through every possible scenario, all of them but the one I was about to hear. Marie told me that Linda, my birth mother, was in a long-term care facility, challenged with Huntington's Disease. Huntington's Disease? What was this? Sitting there, I thought to myself, "Not another disease we don't know about." But then I thought, well, there are three thousand genetic diseases that can be inherited at birth, why not one more?

She said that Mom had been married to the man whose last name we had found on a computerized driver's license list from Hawaii. We knew we had a match and now had to start contacting the family. She gave me the number for my step-father and said the rest was up to me. After some tears, hugs and a prayer, I left and went straight home.

There was a six hour time difference between South Carolina and Hawaii, so I wanted to wait and call when I knew I would get him at home. I had no idea how I was going to approach him and what I was going to say. I did know the Lord had gotten me this far and I knew He would not abandon me. I waited until after his dinnertime, which was after midnight for me. As I was dialing the number, I said, "God, guide my steps and guard my words, place peace in our hearts and keep them open to Your voice and give me Your words."

The warm, kind voice on the other end said, "Aloha."

I proceeded to explain that I was searching for Linda, and wanted to know if he was the gentleman that she had been married to at one point. I also gave enough information so as not to alarm him, but heighten his concern.

"Who are you?" he asked.

"I'm her son." As I uttered those words, the weight on my chest was gone.

I apologized, but he immediately put me at ease and we began discussing everything. It was a shock for him, but a semi-comfortable shock. We began discussing Huntington's Disease. I had no idea of the devastation this disease brings both physically and emotionally, not only for the person challenged, but their entire family. I also learned the disease was able to be passed to the children of the affected person.

As I began to ask a question, he spoke of his children.

"Are your kids my sisters and brothers?" I asked him.

With that, the largest and most comfortable chuckle came from within this tenderhearted bear of a man and he said, "Yes! Yes, they would be! Hold on. I'll go and get them so you can all talk. I think I should tell you one of your sisters and your brother carry the HD gene."

Eventually I talked to my two half-sisters and brother. Each one of them asked me about Huntington's. I didn't know the first thing about it, but was writing quickly and making plans to locate as much information as possible. After a couple of hours on the phone with my new extended family, I knew my search had again begun; this time in a very new direction and with new challenges to face.

After months of communicating and learning about everyone and telling them about me, we started planning the big trip to California. I was going to meet Linda in October. I had spent months learning as much as I could about HD. Comparably, the elation and relief of finding Linda was juxtaposed with the shock and sadness of learning about and accepting this devastating and cruel disease. My concerns about my situation and the possible risk of carrying this disease had become irrelevant, due to my sibling's challenges as well as Mom's.

One afternoon, I found myself a part of a computer List-Serv message board for Huntington's Disease. The number of people and the attitudes overwhelmed me. The sincerity, generosity, and humility these people shared was empowering. I learned more about HD from these wonderfully heroic people on a daily basis than I could from any book or periodical.

Over the next couple of months, I also learned about compassion, acceptance, love, generosity, and faith. Finding myself on the phone too many times to Hawaii, talking with my new sister Kelly, was one of the things that kept my heart at peace and my anxiety at bay. Her sweet, precious voice and tempered demeanor made me feel not only welcome in the family, but bridged the gap of so many years apart. Her vitality, her genuine attention, and her passion for life kept me focused during those first few months. Each time we talked we would discuss HD. Our tones changed every time, but we approached the subject with strength and courage. Kelly had already been a witness to our Mom's progress, and without telling me, I could hear and see how she had been affected.

Through her, I found balance. What impressed me most about Kelly was her love for her family, and especially her love and devotion for her husband, Brian. A sensitive, truly kindhearted man of strength and reserve, Brian supported and attended to Kelly's anticipation of our meeting. I could not be happier and more at peace knowing that Kelly has found her life partner, and what was more important in the coming days was the birth of their first child. Kelly was the spark I needed to refresh my memories of my sister, Clary. Clary died in July of 1988, a month after my fiancée, Jane, died. Just when I thought I would never find anyone like the two most important people in my life, Kelly showed up. A perfect combination of the youth and spontaneity Jane possessed, and the compassion and temperament of Clary. The Lord was working yet another miracle and showing me the circle of life.

July and August brought another new discovery – my other new sister, Stephanie. Married young and already blessed with two beautiful kids, Stephanie helped me recapture that part of my youth that I had been missing. She also helped me see my age and what I had yet to accomplish; the beginning of my own family. Her infectious smile and hearty laughter stirred the joy in me again and, as we got to visit by mail and phone, made me miss a special part of my youth. We had already planned to start trouble when we got together. After all, Mom Linda gave us that gift – the ability to start and carry on good trouble. Our mischievousness is endearing and charming and little did I know what effect we would have on people around us. Stephanie is a strong and committed young woman dealing daily with her genetic rung on the ladder and her baby daughter's. Steph still maintains an incredible, positive, and shining example of hope, something that I needed to find and emulate.

What touched and moved me the most, however, was that I had gained and gotten my life long wish. I had begged Mother and Dad from the youngest age I can remember for a brother. At one point, I even remember yelling at Clary and telling my parents to give her back and swap her for a brother. They laughed, but Clary cried. This really affected me, the sight of her tears. I went to her and said that I loved her and wanted her as my sister but she couldn't be mean to me or she would get sent back in a box. Then she realized the terrorism of her little brother had to change. From then on, we nurtured an intense bond that drew us closer together and that would last until she left us.

The need and desire for a brother, however, didn't dissipate. When Poppa John put Mike on the phone that first night, my heart leaped. I was no longer alone as a man in the family. God had granted my wish years before. A man of strength as well, but a deeply caring and sensitive heart kept Michael very protected and always on guard. The news of my appearance took him by surprise and caused some intense internal feeling. His acceptance and the maturity with which he handled it all was amazing to me. My little brother taught me a great deal about being cool and taking time to let yourself "chill." His light is bright and his sense of humor reflects his inner song. A young man of power still searching for his place in the world was the mirror image I needed to see. My little brother helped save me from self-destruction and pulled me from pain and depression.

My support, education, and ability to relate to my new family came from my new father. Poppa John's warmth, attention, concern and unconditional acceptance consolidated my feelings, fears, and anxiety into a sense of peace and comfort. The first night we all talked, his was the one last voice I heard. After breast cancer took my father in 1991, I longed for that bond that took many years to find. That night on the phone, Poppa John reminded me of Dad, and took over the reins of guidance by calling me, "Son, my other son." Integrity is not something you can buy or be born with. It is acquired and learned from positive experiences, and my life had already been blessed with concrete examples. But these people were beginning to leave me. Poppa John showed up just in time to remind me of my great work and the values I was to base my work on over the next few months. His strength and integrity were powerful, and his smile and laughter made everything easier to accept and handle. His sincerity and frankness when talking about HD was heaven sent. There was no mistaking his heartfelt emotion when talking about HD, but it made acceptance, courage, and determination easier to acquire and to face, fight, and conquer the disease.

The months flew by and all of a sudden I was on the plane to California. On the trip there, I met a wonderful little lady from North Carolina. I sat and shared my story with her. She had been on a Christian retreat of sorts with several friends, one of whom was a birth mother who had recently found her son. As we were preparing to land, she came back to talk to me.

Before leaving, she said something I will never forget. "Listen closely to God's voice, for He will minister and lead you where you need to go, and teach you what you need to learn. Your life is and will be a blessing to others, and you must hold fast to God's knowledge and His salvation, for we can do all things through Christ that strengthens us. You are the gift God gave to your birth mother and she gave you as a gift to your adoptive mother. Your adoptive mother has now given you back to your birth mother so that you can minister to her. God will perform a miracle in her life now through you and your sisters and brother. Never lose sight of how blessed you are for being given these gifts, and never take advantage of God's grace. For through and by His grace you are here doing what He wants you to do, and your needs are being met because this is His will, not yours. Be thankful and bless His name, for the Lord is merciful, His truth is everlasting, and your joy is His gift to you. I hope and pray that you will be a blessing to your families. I know your mother knows that God is leading you; after all, she has helped you search and has sent you on this journey with much love and light and prays for you. And I bless you with love and peace."

Before I could comprehend all of her words, she had kissed my cheek and was on her way back to her seat. I had never heard so many intense words, so deeply felt, from any one person in my life. I had no choice but to listen. That's the way God talks to you sometimes. You have no choice. You have to listen.

All the things you see, emotions you feel when watching a reunion talk show, didn't hold a candle to what those two weeks were like for me. Meeting my new family was an incredible experience, but what changed my life was that first moment I saw her.

I was finally going to meet Linda, my birth mother, for whom I had searched for the better part of my life. I had a good idea of her physical condition, from having read and researched and talked to so many people about HD. I was more than prepared for what I was to see. HD was not going to steal a single second of glory from our reunion. I had witnessed the cruelty of cancer, the devastation of AIDS, the degeneration of Mother's Diabetes, not to mention the other twelve diseases and conditions I had dealt with over the years. Kelly, Stephanie, Mike, and I were all excited and anxious. Coffee had gotten the best of us, especially Mike and me, and we were psyched. We headed out and ended up in several different directions once we got to the mall where we were hunting down last minute gifts and necessities. We finally all made it to the car, and headed to the care center. An awkward silence seemed to drift through the car as we travelled. Between Kelly asking me if I was okay, and Steph and Mike's nervous laughter and carrying on, the ice began to melt. We all began laughing and chattering like kids on the way to Disneyland.

We finally made it to the care center and we piled out of the car. Mike and Steph headed in as Kelly and I brought up the rear. Kelly reached out and gently touched me and said with the most comfortably excited quiet voice, "Are you okay?" I grinned a large "yes" and she said, "Here we go."

While the staff met us, we exchanged pleasantries and the social worker took me back into the center. Mom had been eating her lunch and was in the recreation room. The social worker had found another room a bit more private. I waited outside the room as she went in and prepared Mom for my visit. I could see Linda trying to lean and see me. When the social worker moved to the side, my eyes were transfixed on the most beautiful little lady with the widest eyes and the biggest grin I have ever seen. I went straight to her and as I handed her the flowers I had brought, I watched as one small tear ran down the right side of her face. As it made its salty trail I could feel it intermingling with mine. Through the mist, I embraced her and felt not only her racing heartbeat, but could feel and hear her breathing. All of a sudden, I felt a very shaky and weak arm first touch my side and then up to my shoulder giving me a gentle pat. Linda was saying, in her own special way, "Welcome home, I've been waiting for you."

HD had stolen Linda's ability to speak and her motor and ambulatory skills, but through her excitement and joy, HD took a back seat. Even though Linda could not speak vocally, her eyes contained a library of unread books and

I had opened them all to the first page. Her smile and eyes were fixed on me, and occasionally, she would look over at the social worker and Kelly who was taking pictures for me. I don't know if Mike and Steph were there; I was oblivious to everything else. Our first few minutes together were taken up mostly with me talking to her, and everything I said was coming from an unknown place. Linda was drinking in every word, her eyes reacting to everything I said. Her anxiety as I held her hand and talked to her began to calm, her breathing slowed and her heartbeat began to return to normal. As she hung on to every word, tiny tears trickled down her cheeks. There was no question in my mind that everything I was saying was answering the questions she had had all these years. That wonderful calm we all seek came to Mom and rested on her shoulders like a light spring Carolina snow. We decided that we would go and sit in the parlor area with Mom and visit there.

Being in the care center with so many affected residents was a vivid reminder of all the diseases with which we all contend at times. Alzheimer's, HD, and dementia dominate the make-up of residents, and it was hard to look around. But among all the residents, there was a small group that knew about Linda's long lost son, and they came by the parlor area to squeal and wave and speak. As they did, we all beamed, but Linda brighter than any of us. Her children were together with her and she couldn't have been happier.

God performed a miracle in my life after all those years of searching. I had lived through an unbelievable period in 1988 and 1989. I went through much disease, caregiving and death; all together, ten people and ten traumas in nine short months. I look back on it now as my preparation time for what was to come. I now have two mothers, each ill with their own challenges; one with Brittle Diabetes and one with Huntington's. I am still caregiving and fighting other rampant incurable diseases with which friends are challenged. I am fighting my own demons, but I have a new outlook on life. I have strength, patience, peace, and above all, I have love.

The grave nature of what I witnessed with HD forced me to think of so many questions. Yet, having the strength of spirit and determination to go forward keeps my focus.

The night I spoke to my new stepfather, I learned of my genetic background. Not knowing anything of HD, I was shocked and concerned with the possible risk that I could be faced with in the coming months. Poppa John asked me my age and if I had noticed any of the symptoms. Not having experienced any of them, he seemed to think I might not have the gene, but he still wanted me to know I had an option to be tested.

After our first phone conversation that night, I poured over all the information that I had learned. I remember sitting in my living room that night after my roommate had gone to bed, thinking about all I had finally found. The discovery of my new family was exciting and overwhelming. At this point, I had no choice of what my life may or may not be like. The great question of being tested began to shadow my feelings about the discovery of my new family. Having spent the better part of my life caregiving and watching these diseases take over people's lives, I realized that if this was something I had to deal with in my future, I had to start making plans for security.

The discovery of my risk of HD angered me. I knew it was not Linda's fault, but I felt, "How could the government keep this kind of information from me? How could the Department of Social Services not be required to test babies who are being given up for adoption, for all kinds of genetic and hereditary conditions and diseases?" This, I thought, had to be mandated legislatively. My anger overcame me and the knowledge of my possible risk took what excitement I had and turned it into something negative and depressing.

I began feeling nervous and sad for all of the kids out there who didn't know, and all of the adults like Linda, who had no idea of why they were like they were. My pity, anger, and depression began to turn into strength, hope, and ambition. I was determined to let all the state agencies know what they had kept from my family and me. I knew it was essential to make genetic testing mandatory for all children that were to go through the adoption system. It was the only fair and noble thing for our local government to do.

I also began thinking of how many kids were out there having unprotected sex. With the threat of AIDS and other sexually transmitted diseases (STD's) running rampant among the largest growing infected group, my mind took a turn thinking of the genetic predispositions that could be passed if the young girl involved became pregnant.

I have chosen at this point not to be tested. Kelly and I are of an age, me being older, and we are not experiencing any of the symptoms. I started working towards changing the face of the future by educating whomever I could about the risks, and what the probabilities could be for those who are affected. I also want to send the message out to those unsuspecting people who are considering sharing intimate moments. They need to know that pregnancy and STD's are not the only consequence of unprotected behavior. There are over three thousand genetic diseases, and Huntington's Disease is one of them.

One of my other major concerns involves the medical community and their estimates of who is affected and at-risk from HD. I want to tell them their numbers are way too low. What about all the babies that were adopted out never knowing there was a risk? Aren't they a factor in your numbers, too? I am one of those numbers, but because I was adopted and no one knew, you did not count me.

My concern these days is, of course, assisting in the quest of finding the cure and supporting the families and persons affected by HD. Those who are at-risk and who carry the gene need to know of the dangers, concerns and possible consequences of creating another life, and passing on the risk of this malevolent and unmerciful illness. I feel it my responsibility and priority to educate this group of people. Those of us who were given up for adoption and are at-risk had no choice. But through a commitment to educate, this particular cycle can be broken.

As an adoptee who was born at-risk, I also have a very intense obligation and a vested interest in the legal system concerning National Adoption and Birth Parent Services through the Departments of Social Services and Adoption Legislation. It should be law that this part of our legal system accept and implement the mandatory provision of making medical records concerning genetic disease transmission and heredity available to all parties concerned within the Adoption Triad. Once armed with the knowledge, the war on Huntington's Disease can be won.

Huntington's will only take from us what we give, and allow it to take from us. If we refuse, it will not win. If we fight, it will not win. If we educate, it will eventually lose the battle and it will be eradicated. What a great day that will be. New advances are slowing the grip that this disease takes on the pHD. We are greater and stronger than HD, and it will be cured. There are three things that I take with me each day to remind me that I have a great work to do here before I go on to my eternal home. I have faith in God, unconditional love, and a commitment to shed light.

~ 8

Faces of Family

BY CARMEN LEAL-POCK

Happy or unhappy, families are all mysterious. We have only to imagine how differently we would be described – and will be, after our deaths – by each of the family members who believe they know us.

—Gloria Steinem

I remember an incident when my two sons were about three and four years old. To help you understand, I need to give you our physical descriptions. Although from the mainland, with my brown skin, hair and eyes, I looked more Hawaiian than the locals when we lived on Oahu. My children on the other hand, obviously pulling from their father's German ancestry, were blessed with the most gorgeous blond hair. Once when my oldest son was eighteen months, a woman actually asked me if I dyed his hair. I know I shouldn't have, but the temptation was just too good to pass up. I told her I did, and that I had given him a permanent too, and that was how he got the curls. Worse yet, she believed me.

Along with the blond hair, my younger son has amazing eyes that change from blue to green, and both children have Caucasian features. Back then, people always asked me if they were adopted. Though I usually handled it well and corrected their mistake, sometimes I would have the urge to whip up my shirt and show them my caesarean scars.

On this particular day, I was shopping for that elusive, perfect sofa. They, on the other hand, were wild children. As we travelled from store to store, they jumped on beds, had pillow fights, screamed as loudly as possible and at one store, even burst the festive balloons that announced the grand opening. I was embarrassed, but since I really don't enjoy shopping, I decided I wanted to finish that day and be done with the chore.

The search for the sofa went through lunch and on past nap time. Anyone who has young kids knows that they need to eat and nap on schedule, otherwise everyone pays the price. As their outrageous behavior escalated, people stared and whispered, wondering why I didn't do anything about these ill-behaved children.

My numerous threats and pleadings went unheeded and I decided I'd had enough. I crossed my arms and looked sternly at the boys and said, "This is the last time I will ever baby sit for you again. Wait till I tell your mother just how bad you were." As I continued my tirade, the shoppers nodded their heads in sympathy. Imagine, I was kind enough to take these children, who were obviously not mine, and look how they behaved.

Just as I was bending my arm to pat myself on the back for being so wise and not having to own up to their behavior, my oldest son looked up with his huge chocolate brown eyes and said in that sweet megaphone voice that only kids have, "Mom, how come you're always trying to give us away? Don't you love us?"

Looking at their sweet, cherub like faces, I felt guilty that I had tried to palm the kids off as not mine. What a terrible thing I had done. Not only had I dragged them all over the island and interrupted their schedule, but I had made them feel they were not loved. Without a thought, I gathered them in my arms and we left the store. Shopping was over and if I never got the perfect sofa, at that moment I knew I had the perfect kids.

They say that you can pick your friends, but you can't pick your family. According to Trisha, a member of an HD support group, what that means is, you can't pick your blood relatives but you can surround yourself with friends that become your family. Just like the day my children went wild and I wished I could have two well-behaved children instead of the hellions I had, Trisha says she has often felt that way. "If I had to choose, I would rather not be related to the drug addict aunt and uncle, another alcoholic uncle, or the promiscuous aunt in my family. But I never had any say in the matter and they are in my past and probably in my future."

She goes on to say that she doesn't restrict her family to those who share blood. She considers her close friends family as well. "Since my husband is an only child, and all four of my siblings live in other states, we encourage our three-year-old son to call the friends we care about 'Aunt' and 'Uncle.' I want him to have the support of many relatives, so we create some. I also have had the benefit of a loving family who is not blood. My parents live three thousand miles away and Helen has become like a mother to me. I have a good relationship with my mother, but not like I have with Helen, and her daughter is like a little sister to me. Sometimes close friends can be better than family."

Like many who are married to a spouse with Huntington's, Trisha lives away from her natural family. Helen and her daughter, Tige, helped her paint the entire outside of her house, their only pay gratitude and love. It is these family-friends that we all need to rely on to give us emotional and other types of support.

When I asked the on-line support group what family means to them, the answers were many and varied. Pat answered, "Family is those who commit their lives and their love to each other, even when it hurts. This is the group that lives together, grows together, and dies together." Jeannine had a similar answer. "Family is any person or group of people that create a bond of love, commitment and understanding. I have a large family and they are my blood and I feel a close bond with each one of them, but I also have a few close friends whom I consider family."

Catastrophic diseases like Huntington's can create an even greater need to be surrounded by loved ones. However, the fear and secretiveness that often accompany HD sometimes makes it hard to reach out and ask for support. Just being able to talk about HD is helpful, but even the freedom to do that eludes some people.

Tellie says, "I wish my family was larger. My father has Huntington's and no siblings. He only had two cousins, one died of HD, and the other has relocated, probably in denial. Anyway, there are very few people of my generation and even less in my dad's, so there isn't much discussed or known about HD, except the research I have done. I have two brothers. One is forty, two years younger than me, but he is in denial about HD and will not discuss it rationally. My other brother is only twenty-six and he is the only one who will talk with me about it. We are all concerned about my Dad, who lives alone after being recently widowed. He will not be able to be alone much longer. His mother is still living at ninety-two, but he has nothing to do with her, because he is afraid she will try to force him into religion. We just hope that he gets over this irrational fear, as he has so many others in the past few years. Funny, even very small families can get tied in knots when it comes to HD."

Though she wishes things were different with her siblings and dad, she feels truly blessed by her immediate family because there is a great deal of love and happiness. "My husband of twenty-one years is very supportive," she says. "He just doesn't want to talk about HD too much, either. Our two daughters are fourteen and eight, and I recently informed my oldest about HD being genetic. She took it well, but doesn't really want to talk about it now. We waited until my father was older and we were pretty sure he wouldn't get HD, before having kids. Well, he did have a late onset at about fifty-eight, but we already had the girls by then. I would not trade them for anything, and I would do it again because I feel confident that a cure is right around the corner. I myself have opted to not be tested until the cure is found, or I become obviously symptomatic."

According to Jeannine, "HD has impacted us in both good and bad ways. HD has been a good thing because it makes us realize the importance of today. We say 'I love you' more, we try to laugh harder, live fuller and cry less. HD, or any other terminal illness or major crisis, causes you to re-evaluate what is important in your life. Suddenly, the tiny things that used to be bothersome have just about disappeared. I no longer care whether my house is completely spotless, if it means I can spend an extra hour riding the horse with Scott, or just sitting on the porch watching the stars together. Because later, when Scott is worse, it's the time we spent together that will keep my heart warm."

Of course, there are devastating impacts of Huntington's as well. "The worst part of HD for Scott and I is our decision not to have children," says Jeannine. "It leaves an empty feeling within both of us, but we cope because we know, for us, it's the right decision in our situation. We fill our parental instincts through our three dogs, two cats and one horse. It helps some, but as much as we love our pets, they will never take away the loss of children. The other part that is difficult for me is that I'm losing my best friend in a slow, painful manner, and there's not a thing I can do about it. For Scott, the difficult parts are the loss of independence and self-worth. But even if I had the chance, I wouldn't change anything. I would still have married Scott even if I knew how hard it would be. In fact, I'm thankful for the difficult spots in our marriage because they brought us where we are today. I think finding true love is a special gift, and even though God chose to take so much from both of us, He's also given us so very much in return."

Shirley agrees on the issue of children in an HD family. "If I had known about HD, I probably would not have chosen to have children. But, of course, that is hindsight and cannot be applied to what has already happened. I hate this disease, but I love my sons; they have made me a wiser, kinder person. I learn from them every day; they are my brave heroes and I will do what I can to make their lives better. They have made our entire family closer, more loving and patient."

Families can sometimes come about as a result of what some people consider different circumstances. Teri tells her story and how the shape of her family changed for the better. "I met my stepmother Barbara when I was only eight. By then, my mother was very sick with Huntington's Disease. At first, I wasn't too sure about Barb, because Mom was still alive and Dad was still married to her. My dad introduced Barb to the family. Of course,

Mom was confused at first, but I guess she realized that Dad needed help raising two kids. Many people disagree with what happened next, and I certainly understand why they would disagree. But to an eight-year-old, change was going to happen and I guess it was better that it was a positive change. After a time, my dad divorced my mom and married Barb. All five of us moved into a bigger house together. Barb was only twenty-two at the time and became the caregiver for Mom, and a stepmom to Sheri and me. She did everything for my mom. She fed her, bathed her, took her for walks and talked to her. Mom and Barb became pretty good friends and she cared for Mom at home until we had to place her in nursing home. As the disease progressed, Mom started getting up in the middle of the night and falling and hurting herself. I can't count the times Dad and Barb spent the night in the E.R. getting Mom stitched up. Even after Mom went into the nursing home, we all, as a family, went to see her every Sunday. My dad went daily, but that Sunday was family time and that included Barb."

Teri goes on to explain, "Barb and Dad eventually had two more children of their own. Barb was amazing; she took care of her two little ones, my sister Sheri, and me. She was in the New Mexico Symphony Orchestra, was in a private quartet, and went to college. How she did all this, I have no idea but I am so grateful that she did. Dad has always been a workaholic so I don't know how we would have made it without Barb. She is definitely my family, my hero and my guardian angel. We are still extremely close and I love her very much."

Sometimes the effects of HD can be devastating to families. Two years ago a man from Hunt-Dis tested positive for HD. Since that time, his wife couldn't handle the results and the way he treated her, so now she is no longer in his life. As he describes what he is going through, he says, "The pain and hurt this has brought on is unbearable. I wonder every day when something happens, something drops, or I can't remember things. Is this the start of HD? It's like living under a microscope. The depression and the feeling of being alone through this ordeal is overwhelming. People need to be thankful for each and every day God gives them to work, play and enjoy their spouses and children. Never take any of them for granted, because life is so uncertain, we never know what we have until it's gone." For him to be diagnosed as having the gene and then to suffer the agony of divorce was very painful. But even in the midst of this, or possibly because of this, he finds strength in other places. "My only strength to go on comes from getting really centered with God and asking Him for more time, and thanking Him for the time I do have. I also thank Him for all the wonderful people this ordeal has brought into my life. He does ease the pain and hurt if you let Him in. I have three children and the guilt that I might have passed this on to them is great. I did not know about my father having the gene until after all were born. He came back into my life by a phone call thirty-seven years after leaving."

Kathy eloquently describes her life, her struggles as a child in a family with an HD parent.

> "The struggle to maintain a career, be a loving spouse and companion to an increasingly demented woman, and to provide all that the children needed was my father's. The struggle to understand a deranged mother and grow into healthy, strong adults was my sibling's and mine. The struggle to cope with ever diminishing abilities and hold on to as much of precious life as possible

was my mother's. It may be helpful for you to know, though, that my brother, sister, and I left that home with strength, character, commitment, bravery, and insight way beyond our years. We lived with a bizarre mom and a tirelessly and humorously devoted father. He shared his struggles and everything he knew about my mom's disease with us, and we learned about commitment, patience, finesse, failure, persistence, anger, kindness, and faith; and a little bit of genetics and neurology for good measure. As my husband and I face the same fate since I have tested positive, our challenge is to meet this piece of our destiny with even greater success than my father. I hope that we are up to it."

Families with Huntington's Disease are no different than others in many ways. There are those that are loving and supportive, lone individuals, and everything in between. Regardless of whether we are talking about our blood relatives or people we have grown to care about, we all need to be a part of something greater than ourselves.

Susan Garrett is HD positive. "I am also a single parent of two children," she said. "I get tired so easily now. Before, I could stay up late, get up early and be fine. Now every thing I do is a real struggle. I work full time and worry every day about what we will do when I can't work any more, as I am the sole supporter for my family. I feel very, very overwhelmed and scared of my future. Though I am going through all of this, I am glad for my life. I am glad that I am working at a good job with supportive people and I belong to a wonderful church that is filled with love and support. Without this support, I don't know what I would do. Last weekend, a group of young men from our church came over and cleaned up my yard and got me in good shape to face the upcoming spring and summer. The hardest part of all of this is to be on the receiving end of things. I would rather be on the giving end."

Susan is blessed in how her family handles HD and she has wise words to share.

"No one understands what it is like to be in our shoes until they have been there. Luckily, in my family, they have not hidden HD from us, but embraced it; we pulled closer together because of that bind. My father died of HD, but we have a reunion with his family every two years. The love that is felt there is so strong. Some have HD, some think they might, others have received a happy negative test. But, even with the good results, it is still our entire family's problem to handle. My sister, just older than me at forty-eight, is symptomatic, and recently had to be moved back home to live with my mom because she can't take care of herself. She has been a great inspiration to me. When she first found out she had HD, she was sad and cried lots of tears. After that, she set her mind that she was going to enjoy every minute of every day. She has handled this much better than I have. I am still fighting it. Two other siblings who have been tested are negative. They both felt guilty when they got their results and told me that they didn't have total relief because of my sister and me. Both have gone out of their way to help us and support us through our struggles. I have one more sister who has not been tested yet. She is raising a beautiful family of six kids and feels that is all the stress she can have in her life right now."

She continued to share about another situation. "In the support group, one lady said that everyone in her family that had HD killed themselves. She even tried to do it to herself. She lived and was very angry. She said she told

God that He had better make her life worth living if she was going to have to live through this. She started coming to the support group, met a man there with HD, and they got married. Even though every time I see them they are physically getting worse, they tell me that life does go on and we should make the most of every moment. Another lady in our support group told us that her entire family disowned her when they found out she had HD. There are so many stories out there. Some families are supportive, like mine, and others are hiding it. It is so very hard for everyone involved."

∽

Mother

BY GABRIELLE HAMILTON

You are not listening to me
as I try to make your life easier
   by assuming more
   and more of your burdens
like, I thought
   you wanted me to do.

Though thirty seconds before
   you were smiling
   and laughing
I am now suffering
   your rage and anger
as though you can't stand
   the sight of me
and wished I'd just go away.
No matter how hard I try
   to explain myself

I know that the cacophony in your head
        won't let you hear me
        as you once would have.
I feel your frustration
        whirl around me –
like a dust storm –
        until my eyes water and tear
and the arrogant indifference in your eyes
        forces me to quell the sob
still in my chest.
I wonder if you realize
        that you are no longer who you once were.
She listened and loved completely
        while you are conditional and self-absorbed.
You are fortunate that
        I remember her
enough to care about you
and I am fortunate to have known her.

March 26, 1995

∾

Leo's Story

BY LEO WAYNE PIKE

In 1946, when I was twelve, I watched my mother die of Huntington's Disease. She died in a State Hospital in Peoria, Illinois. In those days, it was not uncommon for a person with Huntington's Disease to be placed in an institution.

My dad had died when I was even younger, so I stayed alone with my mother before she was institutionalized. I had older twin brothers and two sisters, but I was living at home alone with my mother in this condition until, finally, one day I confronted my older brothers with the fact that this could not go on. After that, my mother was hospitalized, and she never returned home again.

At that time, I did not know what was happening. I had never heard of Huntington's Disease. My mother's movements all her waking hours were involuntary. Yet, I used to see her asleep and wonder why she could lie there so quietly with no symptoms of this disease. It is hard for anyone to watch a person they love fall apart even when they know why it is happening. It was difficult for such a young man as I was to live with the effects of this horrifying disease.

Later, as she and I worked in a business running an amusement park, I observed my beautiful sister wither away to nothing. She too had been stricken. My twin brothers did not escape either. Lamar began showing symptoms in 1965, and died of Huntington's in a Veteran's Hospital in Danville, Illinois. The other, Clyde, had a heart attack at age fifty-seven. I now know that Clyde no doubt had Huntington's Disease, as they were identical twins.

My mother died at the age of fifty. As far as I can remember, it seemed as if it was about fifteen years from the onset until she passed away. My sister Bernice showed symptoms in her late thirties, and she died when she was fifty-eight years old.

I did a lot of genealogy research tracing my family, trying to find out where this dreadful disease had originated. I was able to discover that my grandfather on my mother's side died of Huntington's Disease in a State Hospital in Kentucky. After I visited the facility, they sent me to the archives that were stored in Frankfurt, Kentucky, where the records showed his admission into the hospital, his diagnosis and death.

Support group meetings I attended were helpful with suggestions for people who had family members affected by Huntington's Disease, which I did. I had some relatives who were at-risk for HD and they decided to live their lives in the extreme. Maybe they were afraid of HD and wanted to make the most of their time before it was too late.

As for me, it never bothered me whether I would contract HD or not. I can't explain it, but I just wasn't concerned. I never used HD as an excuse for going off the deep end and I have lived a normal life. I went into the service when I was eighteen years old... World War II, of course. I married a wonderful Christian woman when I was twenty-one who deserves all the credit for guiding me and keeping me on an even keel. We have two children, and I never gave the fact that we had Huntington's Disease in our family a thought. I guess I was ignorant about the disease. It was through my wife's effort that I became knowledgeable.

As it turned out, at the age of seventy I can say I have escaped the disease, and therefore, my children and grandchildren will not contract Huntington's. If I had known more about the consequences of Huntington's, I may not have had children. What a blessing it is that I didn't know, because I have two wonderful and talented children and four granddaughters. As far as I know, there weren't any tests for Huntington's then. My sister, who died from Huntington's Disease, also had two children. One of her daughters was into drugs and alcohol and she died in an automobile accident in her thirties. The other daughter, Diane, died of diagnostic MS. Sometimes, I wonder if it had some connection with Huntington's.

To my knowledge, there are no other family members who are showing signs of Huntington's, although several are still at-risk.

You Are Always There

BY KELLY ELIZABETH MILLER

When I got into trouble, you were always there.
And when I got into fights, you were always there.
And when I had a fall to drugs, you were always there.

You know all of my faults, but you still stay.
I've hurt you so many times, but you're still always there.
I've put you through so much sorrow and pain
and over a million times I have disgraced your name.
But still again, you were always there.

Why? I don't know. But each day you teach me more,
as you've done in the past.
And if anyone ever asks me to describe the word "love,"
I would say truly and honestly, "My Mother."

FACES OF HUNTINGTON'S

"I Will Always Love You"
BY BRENDA PARRIS SIBLEY

Sitting in your chair
in the nursing home,
you hold my hand,
but you barely respond.
You can't understand me;
I can't understand you.
Words have no meaning.
Neither do faces.
You've been on the way
here for a long time.
But did I speed it up?
In trying to care for you,
did I do more harm than good?
And then I gave up,
and now you just sit.
Mama, I'm so sorry.
Mama, I'm so afraid
that I did this to you.

January 1996, copyright © 1996

What I Wish

BY ANDREA HADDIX

Having a parent with Hu[…]
hard. My heart aches for an[…]
that's not much help in and […]
that situation. You see, I lived[…]
my sisters having this terrible[…]

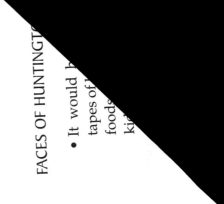

I detested, and felt such guilt that we had to leave Daddy in the veteran's home and hospital, and hated that we had to place my sister in a residential care facility just a few years later. I vowed then that if anybody else got sick, I would move mountains to do my all so that I wouldn't have any reason to feel guilt. It's almost slavish this fear I have, but I just want to love my family members even more... it's like an unexpressed essence that wants to burst my heart wide open. It's pain turned into love that must flow out. That's what it is.

You know what I wish? I wish my dad hadn't withdrawn as he did. Even though others thought he looked funny, to me he was the handsomest, most wonderful man in all the world. See, Andi, the kid, did not know how to talk to Dad like Andi, the grown up, wishes she could have. I have all these missing pieces; all these unsaid "I love you's," all these unspoken interactions, and I can't fix it. I don't have many pictures, we have no movies or videotapes, no tapes of him talking, and no letters from him.

I have a list of things that I wish we had done when I was a kid that would help me today and would have helped me then.

- I wish we had taken home movies of Dad and us kids interacting.

145

...ave been wonderful if Dad had made
...his thoughts... about politics, sports, favorite
..., music, what he liked best about each of us
...us (because we were all different and unique and
...special).

- Oh, if we had only taken lots of pictures of Dad and us kids together.
- We should have made things together that would have endured time.
- I wish we had written letters to Dad and he to us.
- We needed to make memories, any way we could have.

I have to remember that even though it was hard to see my dad sick, the kid that I was still loved Dad with my whole heart. If I have to hate anything at all, I hate the disease, not my dad.

Anyway, I wanted more from my dad than he could give at the time. We were all so shell-shocked, with no support from any outside source whatsoever, that we couldn't even begin to think of things to do to make it better. It was strictly survival mode. Absolutely.

I guess when you have knowledge that you are gene positive, it would seem the responsible and prudent thing to abstain from having children. Your children will suffer from HD... whether they are positive or negative. HD is who we are, regardless.

Waiting For the Next Chapter

BY DONNA T. DUFFY

On January 23, 1991, my sister, Bonita (Bonnie) Krummel, disappeared. There is not a day that passes that I don't wonder where she could be. I find it difficult to believe she destroyed herself, though some say she did just that. If it is so, the killer was Huntington's Disease.

When my grandmother died in 1953, at the age of fifty-three, an autopsy was done to discover the reason for her death. It revealed a diagnosis of Huntington's Disease. Unfortunately, by the time her four children reached their mid-thirties to early forties, each one of them had developed definite HD symptoms.

In all, there were eight offspring from the four children. When we were young, it was difficult to understand our parents' strange behavior, but we were never allowed to ask questions about it. But I knew something not very pleasant was happening in our family. I just prayed it wouldn't happen to me.

My Uncle Marcy would just start screaming and lock himself in the bathroom until we left the house. His oldest son, Robert, seems fine, but Jeanette is already in a nursing home at age forty-five. My Aunt Teddy tried to commit suicide twice, and each time she has failed. I don't know if her sons Charles and Louis have escaped their mother's fate. My Aunt Nancy also tried to commit suicide and failed, but her sons Philip and Nicky seem to be free from the HD sentence.

My mom continually screamed about anything and everything. For two years, she was so distressed that alcohol became her best friend. Of course, that brought on a complete other set of problems. She did become a little quieter then, but she was still embarrassing; we could never have a friend over for fear of what she might do next. She was both physically and emotionally destructive, and though I could fill pages with examples, I won't because I have tried so hard to bury the hurt inside.

When I was sixteen, my father told my sister and me that our mother had Huntington's Disease, but I still did not associate her behavior with a physical illness. She had tormented me so much, I can honestly say I had developed a hatred for her. I would have given anything to have what I considered a real a mom, and not "that person" hurting me more with each passing day. It got so bad sometimes that my mother and I would have fist fights. Afterwards, she would be sweet, changing completely, and I would feel guilty about the fights.

These were not easy times, and years later, watching my sister trying to handle this disease, I finally came to terms with my past. I realized that part of my mother's anger and actions were caused by HD.

Bonnie first began to notice symptoms in 1984. She was a pleasant person, docile by nature, and never had anything bad to say about anyone, since she accepted people the way they were. Though she never got as bad as my mother, with the onset of HD she screamed a lot and made many uneasy movements. Her two children, Keith and Kirsten, now eighteen and fifteen, had no idea their mother was sick until she disappeared. Yes, they knew she was different from other mothers in some ways, but they figured that was just the way she was. My mother was hospitalized in 1978, so they could never relate the HD symptoms their grandmother had to those their mother was experiencing.

Because my sister dealt with HD by not talking about it, she thought the only people who knew were her husband, Cardin, my husband, and me. This simply was not true. Everyone who knew our family history believed she had inherited the gene, but they loved and respected her enough not to mention it.

By October of 1990, I knew my sister had to talk to someone. Bonnie was holding all her fears, anger, and emotions inside. When I suggested she see a psychologist, she became angry and said she could not talk to people as I could. I called her neurologist before my sister went to the appointment and asked the doctor to suggest that Bonnie see someone on a professional level to discuss what was happening to her; the doctor said she could not discuss Bonnie's case with me. I explained I didn't need to "discuss" the case at all. I had lived with HD all my life and knew more than any doctor could possibly know. I just wanted Bonnie to get help.

The neurologist did suggest that Bonnie see a psychologist, but of course, she quickly refused and the conversation moved on to other things. She walked out with a prescription for Haldol, the same medication given to my mother twenty years prior. I was not happy because I had seen what it had done to my mother. The doctor did not tell her that two of the possible side effects of the drug were depression and sleeplessness. All she explained was that it would lessen the terrible movements.

At first, Bonnie appeared calmer, but by Christmas, I knew the medication was not helping; Bonnie's movements were rapid and she was quite nervous. As much as I wanted to discuss her symptoms with her, I knew this was not the proper moment for it. I was also going through my own mental anguish at the time, as I was awaiting the results from my six months pre-symptomatic testing for Huntington's Disease. Originally, I was to hear the results before Christmas, but because of a communications error, I had to wait until January 11.

The negative results I received left me thrilled, yet hesitant to tell Bonnie. I finally got the courage to tell her at 4:00 in the afternoon. I was frightened by her possible reaction, and I felt guilty; I still do in many ways. We'd been so close and had shared every aspect of our lives. I got mixed emotions about telling her that I'd been spared her fate because I thought she would feel even more frightened and alone. To my amazement, Bonnie did not even respond to my announcement. Instead, she began chattering about a store going out of business. I did not know how to react so I just continued on with her conversation.

On January 26, 1991, Bonnie was planning a dinner party for some friends. Three days before the party, she called me and asked that I cancel the party. She told me she had not slept in four nights and wasn't functioning well. Her chorea only stopped when she slept, so her body never got a chance to rest. On top of the natural stress of sleep deprivation and HD, Bonnie had finally told her mother and father-in-law that she had the disease. Though it was a relief to let them know, it probably increased her nervousness.

The neurologist prescribed an anti-depressant, but her weary body still did not get rest that night. When Bonnie called again, she was told to increase the dosage to two pills, but it was never suggested she might want to come in to see the doctor. Bonnie hated taking medication, and taking the second pill, which didn't seem to help, threw her over the edge. I told Bonnie I would cancel the party for her.

After Bonnie and I spoke, she and Cardin went to the mall to return something and then stopped at the store to buy lunch, which they brought home. During that time, Cardin says Bonnie was quiet. When Keith and Kirsten came home from school, Bonnie was at the kitchen table doing her nails and staring out the window. She may have been contemplating something all day, but no one will ever know for sure.

At 2:45 p.m., she announced that she was going out for a little while. Cardin asked if he should take her, but she said no. He backed the car out for her and told her not to leave the town where they lived. He also reminded her that Kirsten had to pick up Girl Scout cookies and go to a skating party that night.

Driving was quite unsafe for Bonnie because of her movements, but taking away someone's freedom is difficult. She had recently had two car accidents, and Cardin was understandably uncomfortable whenever she drove. He was, of course, concerned when she had not returned by dinner time, but carried on as usual, taking the children out to eat and afterwards dropping Kirsten off for the party. When Kirsten returned from skating, Bonnie was still not home.

At 9:00, Cardin called and informed me that Bonnie had left the house in the afternoon and had not returned. We discussed the possibility that she had gone to the mall and lost track of time. Though this was not typical of Bonnie, by this time we were trying not to panic and willing to assume anything.

At 9:45, Cardin could not wait any longer; he called the police to explain the situation. They arrived shortly thereafter to take down whatever information that Cardin could give them. At 11:00, the police called me to ask whether I had heard from my sister and other important questions. I asked if I should come to the station, but they suggested I stay home in case Bonnie called and wanted to talk. It was the roughest night my family and I have ever been through.

At 6:00 the following morning, I called Cardin and he told me Bonnie's car had been found at 12:45 a.m., parked in front of the library, not far from their home. Bonnie was nowhere to be found. By 7:00, I was on my way to their house with my daughter, never having received a call from my sister.

Inside the car was Bonnie's handwritten note that read, "I am sorry that it had to come to this, but I can't go on another minute. I love you all. Love, Bonnie." She also left the jewelry she was wearing in the console, and her pocketbook was slightly stuffed under the driver's seat. Everything was still in the pocketbook – wallet, glasses, charge cards, license, and other personal effects.

This was the beginning of the nightmare. The police had responded quickly in the most crucial hours when my sister was reported missing. They searched every hospital, morgue and shelter, along with contacting every store owner, employee or patron who might have been in the stores my sister was in the night she disappeared. All the people in my sister's telephone book were called, bus drivers were questioned, and the car was finger printed.

A police dog came in to pick up Bonnie's scent that led the police to the lake in the park, but police divers came up empty handed. A second dog was brought to the house, and again the scent was to the lake. The police dredged the lake, but again, nothing was found.

The nightmare has never ended; the mystery of my sister is still unsolved. There is not one hour I do not think of her. I feel so incomplete. The emptiness is impossible to explain, because my sister was a very important part of my life. She was always there for me since the time I was little, until the day she disappeared, and sometimes I even forget she is gone, and have a strong need to share with her.

Whenever there is news of a body being found, I pray that this could be it. I may know in my heart she is gone, but I need someone to tell me they have her body. Only then can I rest.

I love Bonnie with all my heart and soul. I understand that Huntington's Disease caused her to do what she did. I just need a final word to end this chapter of my life.

∽

A Mother's Love

BY SHIRLEY PROCELL

The magic of morning
Damp blades of grass
Bright colored flowers
None of these last
The love of a Mother
Is here and will stay
Getting stronger and stronger
With each passing day
The morning soon fades
Grass and flowers will die
But the love of a Mother
Is always nearby
She stands beside you
Again and again
Her love's unconditional
And will last to the end.

A House Divided

BY MONTSE TORRECILLA

There was never a time I can remember when my aunt wasn't sick. My mother's sister just didn't act normal. Her behavior was strange and my mother always seemed to say, "Don't bother your aunt, she is sick."

My aunt, her husband, and their four daughters lived three hundred kilometers from us. We used to visit them three or four times a year, and with every trip, my aunt seemed to worsen. I can still remember her sitting in a chair, without speaking, her bright blue eyes trying to catch what was around her, smiling crazily. Later in her bed, I saw her blue eyes, vacant, not trying to catch anything anymore.

For many years, she was just someone suffering from a mental disease, schizophrenia or hysteria, it seemed. Later, after she tried to commit suicide, doctors found that she had a neurological problem, but she never did get diagnosed with Huntington's Disease.

When I was expecting the first of my children, Maria, my oldest cousin, Conchita, began having some strange symptoms. None of the doctors she visited thought it had anything to do with her mother's problems. She was young and she was quickly deteriorating. They first said she had Friederick's Ataxia, but after a while, the doctors confirmed that she had HD. With that diagnosis, we all assumed that her mother had the same sickness.

Life continued, with the disease not touching us at all. We seemed far removed from the drama being played out in my aunt's family. Now, I can't understand how my own family could have been so naive.

I was expecting my fourth and last child when my mother began having symptoms that I immediately recognized as those that Conchita had at the beginning. Since my mother was sixty-seven years old, the doctors determined that yes, she had mental deterioration, but not due to any disease. My mother, they said, was just suffering from the normal aging process. We insisted it was more than that, so one doctor ordered a series of tests, including an MRI. They finally agreed it could be more than age, but they were still not willing to concede it was HD.

Somehow, I knew that my mother had HD, but I wanted to be sure. Back then, the only test you could perform was one that required blood samples from different members of the family. I couldn't find anyone who wanted to cooperate with me for the test because none of my cousins wanted to know anything about HD. They were completely afraid and so they preferred the comfort that comes from forgetting a problem exists. Finally, I had to admit defeat at trying to get my family to help, but I never let go of the fact that I knew this disease could one day affect us.

By then I had four children and I knew that until I was sure if I had the disease or not, they too were at-risk. Of course, my family never considered this was a problem that could affect us. I began to panic when I thought of my children. I always thought I was a clever person, how could I have had four children without considering the wisdom of that since I knew there was obviously something wrong in my mother's family?

Two years ago, we switched my mother to a new doctor. After one examination, he was sure that it was HD, but wanted to confirm it with the new test. The discovery of the gene in 1994 made the need to test other family member's blood obsolete.

While we waited for the results of the test, I tried to get all the information I could about this disease. In Spain, there was virtually nothing written about Huntington's

Disease and so I turned to the Internet. Although there was nothing in Spanish, I did have enough knowledge of English to be happily impressed and relieved when I found so much information. What I thought was a forgotten disease, unknown and affecting only a few people, was completely different. I signed onto the on-line support group called Hunt-Dis, and my education really began. I have been a member of this group since its inception, and have been in contact with hundreds of people like myself, who were beginning to understand more about Huntington's. As I learned about this disease, I became less afraid of it, but I was sure that I wanted to know if HD was going to affect my children and me.

Six months after her blood was drawn, we got my mother's results; she had tested positive for the gene with thirty-eight CAG repeats. Once I heard the news, I decided I, too, wanted to take the test, and the doctor agreed. Amazingly, only one day after learning of my mother's positive results, the testing process began. Unlike in other countries, there was no requirement for a neurological examination, no psychological interview or any counseling. I told my only sister what I was going to do, and she told me I was crazy. I told my husband and he asked me, "Why?" Why was I so obsessed with HD? Why did I want to know? Wasn't it better simply to let time go on? What difference could knowing make?

But I needed to know because I wanted to be able to plan my future. I was willing to live with fear if there was a reason, but I didn't want to dread something that possibly didn't exist. I was sure that I had symptoms and that I had inherited the HD gene. I was so much like my mother and saw similarities at every turn. I felt I could handle either result, I just wanted to live as full a life as possible, one way or the other. I became obsessed with knowing and I think one of the reasons was my husband. One year earlier, my husband was diagnosed with cancer of the larynx and had his vocal cords and larynx removed. He had no problems after surgery and the doctors assured him they had removed all cancer cells. But he was only forty-one years old and it was not easy to go on after that. If I was going to be touched by some disease, I wanted to know so I could plan and live a very good life. And I was, of course, concerned for my four children. If I had the gene, we needed to plan for their future.

I knew from the Hunt-Dis list that in the United States, you had to see many doctors before having the test. I thought how wonderful it was not to have to go through anything at all. The only thing the neurologist asked me before the test was, if the result was positive, would I agree to visit a psychiatrist. Of course, I said yes.

In May 1996, I got the results; I was negative. I couldn't believe it; I still can feel this happiness inside me. I have never been so happy and I know I'll never be again. I sat down with my beautiful children and explained everything to them. I had wanted to shield them from uncertainty, so they never heard a word about HD and they were surprised, but also happy. Even the small one, at five years old, understood that something very important had happened to all of us. No one except my father, my sister and my husband knew about my decision to get tested, but I phoned my cousins to tell them. They congratulated me and I know they were sincere and happy for me. I told my parents-in-law and they were happy. I told my father and of course he felt relieved. Only my sister acted distant and seemed as if she was not very pleased with the result. Although she first said it was good news and she was happy about my results, something happened, and from that moment, our relationship changed.

She became more distant and rejected any contact with me. I tried to get closer to her, but she would always pull away. After some time had passed, she told me that I had hurt her profoundly. It seems this was because I had told some friends and my in-laws about my results, without thinking that she wasn't tested yet, and she could have inherited the HD gene.

I could not believe what I was hearing. Now, after over a year, I understand what she felt, but not then. I was so happy that I could not help telling my closest friends or my husband's family the reasons for this happiness. I never thought that my new status would hurt my sister, and that our relationship would become so badly damaged.

Eventually, my sister too decided to take the test to determine her future. Unlike my joy, her testing produced in her a sadness, as she received a positive result. She did it without telling my father or me. I only learned of her testing and subsequent results because eventually she told my father, and he told me, although he had promised to keep the news a secret from me. She went through the testing as I did; no neurological exams, no psychologist, no counseling, and now I know why the entire testing process is so important. I am convinced that if she had gone through all the counseling, she wouldn't have been allowed to continue. Now, she is alone. Her husband is a beautiful person and I am sure he will take care of her, but he is not the kind of person someone can cry with or explain their tears to.

She knows I am involved with HD and that I have a lot of information, but she refuses to accept anything from me or to learn about Huntington's. I would like to tell her that it is not my fault that she is positive while I am negative. I would like to tell her that I am here for whatever she wants, that I am not against her but with her. But she doesn't want to listen, or maybe right now she cannot. I hope as time goes on, things will change and we can be friends again. That is my sincere wish, but right now, being as stubborn and hurt as she is, that seems impossible.

The worst of it all is that we are not the only family in which this has happened. I know that in many HD families, situations such as these happen, and it is terrible. In our case, my mother somehow can sense the void between her two daughters, but does not understand the explanation. The rift that has been created is hard on everyone, at a time when we should be helping each other.

Although I was blessed with a negative result, I will never abandon the HD cause. I feel I have to fight in the only way I can; by getting information to the people who need it, or just trying to let people know they are not alone. There is not a great awareness of HD in Spain, so just telling people that HD exists is a big job. It is a job I will do for the rest of my life.

Dear Child

By Jeannine Dutton

Dear child I won't conceive,
I am sorry for the warmth of your tiny soul,
Which I will not feel.
I love you more than to have you,
For I know the cramped dark corner,
From which you would be forced to grow.
I have tasted the sourness,
From whence you may fall.
I cherish you more.
So, I let you remain a flower,
To grow within my mind,
Safe among the green grasses.

I could not bear to witness,
Your birth as a tender flower,
The needing to adapt into a bitter weed,
Only to grow up in between,
The concrete called disease.
Yet, even the stalk of the bitter weed,
Might not withstand,
The frozen draft of this peril.
You could wither,
And even leave a seed or two.
To your father's eyes so blue.
He wants you badly, too.

Easy I make our choice seem,
Loftily I dodge questions posed,
Casually toss my head and turn.
But dear one,

There is not a sun that rises,
Without an ache for you,
For I know the love you would bring,

But, wise I need to be,
For I have witnessed this disease,
Turn eyes of tenderness,
Into flints of rage and fear.
I have seen the madness,
Cause one to wish for death,
And grant the wish himself.
I have watched a struggle,
With demons that would be your future.
I have wiped helpless tears,
Cried for lost childhood,
And caressed sadness,
That erodes the landscape of life.
I love you more than to have you.

The Wild Plant

BY ELTON D. HIGGS

Some seeds we plant
Grow counter to
The cultivator's plan.

No vision can encompass
What may spring from
Sun and water, ground and care –
What flowers there defy
The formal garden
Laid out to please the mind.
This kind of flower
Grows uncomfortably
Past the bed that
Incubated it, wrestles
With the order of its inception.

And in its turn
It seeks to propagate
The license of some
Unknown and wild progenitor;
While I, poor ordered I,
Can only clip a tendril
Here and there,
And share the way God's love
Entwines and sweetens
Even bitter herbs.

Memories of Dad

BY MARY EDWARDS

My dad was the light in my world. He was what all daddies should be.

My dad was the one who joined his daughters and their friends when we sneaked out of bed to have ice cream during our slumber party. He laughed so much at our silliness that he woke up my mom.

He said he liked chrysanthemums, but would never say the word because he could never tell when he was finished. He added syllables to the word till we never knew when it would end. Chrysanthemum-mum-mum-mum-mum-mum.

My dad called my Annette "Princess" all her life and made her feel like one too.

Daddy is responsible for my divorce because I thought all men were like him but I have lived long enough to know that there are NO men like him. He really had nothing to do with my divorce, but I used to tease him about it.

He always said my mother had "gone to er" when she was having her hair done; as in, "She is always pretty; she goes to get pretti-ER."

When my mom had a stroke, he said, "She is not exactly my Ruth anymore, but I'll take her any way I can get her. And he did, until he died shortly before their fifty-fourth wedding anniversary.

My dad always told me I could do anything I wanted to, if I wanted it enough. He gave me so much, so often, in such a gentle, loving fashion. He is my prescription for the world.

My friends used to "borrow" him from time to time. I hope that you will smile a little at my silly, wonderful, loving dad. If you want to, you can borrow him too.

Stories of Fear, Stories of Love

BY CARMEN LEAL-POCK

When my husband was first diagnosed with Huntington's Disease, I tried to find available information about what we were facing. Eventually, I found a checklist in a pamphlet where various symptoms were listed. It looked a little like the list below.

Characteristics/Symptoms:

Personality changes, depression, mood swings, unsteady gait, involuntary movements, slurred speech, impaired judgment, difficulty in swallowing, intoxicated appearance

I have since learned that not every person with HD has every symptom. My husband has very little chorea, mainly twitching in his hands and feet. His swallowing and behavior changes are significant and cause the majority of his problems. It is important to treat each pHD as an individual, as there is no one blanket-treatment for HD. It is often a series of trial and error.

The symptoms that can be most disturbing and dangerous are those relating to behavior. One of the reasons I was attracted to my husband Dave was because of his gentle, loving personality. He never raised his voice and seemed to have an infinite amount of patience. With the onset of HD, he seemed to change overnight. The sharp words and unreasonable expectations soon escalated to uncalled-for rages.

Once, Dave left the room where he was watching television. My younger son, then twelve years old, not knowing Dave had been sitting in a specific chair, sat down to watch the program. Out of nowhere, Dave flew at my son, cursing at him for being in the chair. Dave picked him up, threw him against the wall, and began beating him with his cane. When I tried to intervene, he turned on me with increased fervor until, finally, he stopped, walked outside into the rain and stood on the street crying. That is when I knew we needed help. I am so thankful that we were able to find a medication that helped to relieve the severity of those symptoms so we could all remain in the household.

No, every person with HD does not turn into a monster. But it is important to know that it could happen and that it is the disease and not the person. Often, even before diagnosis or other symptoms appear, outbursts and inappropriate behavior can create a dangerous environment for the person suffering with HD and others as well. Families, especially, are vulnerable to the behavior issues, be it from a spouse, a parent, or a child.

In collecting stories for this book, I have heard countless family members describe the horror of living with someone who literally seems to become a new, dangerous person. The mental, verbal, and physical abuse in some cases has torn families apart. This is not an easy subject to talk about. However, having been subjected to unexplainable rage and violence by my normally easygoing husband, I have to believe others are going through the same type of thing.

Yes, HD gives a reason for the behavior, but it is still not acceptable. Today, there are effective medications to successfully treat personality changes, depression, and mood swings. In the booklet, "A Physician's Guide to the Management of Huntington's Disease – Pharmacologic and Non-Pharmacologic Interventions," available from the HDSA, the "outbursts" are discussed. Whether a pHD is prone to easy anger and now they rage directly at their targets with the smallest provocation, or is slow to anger and have "occasional outbursts," they can be controlled by environment and/or medication.

I wish this chapter on families was one hundred percent warm and fuzzy and each story shared was about how the disease has made them realize just how much they love each other. In most cases, that is true. But I have tried to draw many faces of Huntington's even when the faces are hurtful and cause pain and tears. Two women, whose names are withheld, have graciously allowed me to tell a tiny bit of their stories. If you recognize yourself or someone you love in these words, please do whatever is necessary to get help.

Always in Fear

Once, when my husband was in one of his rages, he put my arm out of commission for several weeks. I went to the doctor, but I never told him what happened, just asked him to fix it. There have been so many rages with this disease. My husband told our family doctor, while my daughter and I were there, that his behavior was "perfectly appropriate for the situations." Normal?

Writing this brings back painful memories and it is not particularly fun to bare my soul like this. So many times I have wanted to talk to others about what my family has experienced; others who might be suffering the same emotional and physical abuse that I did because of Huntington's Disease. I would love nothing more than to shove those memories and experiences deep in back where they would never see the light of day. That's the easy thing to do. But if it's helpful to someone else, I have been there and am willing to support the next person in any way that I can.

There was a time, ten years ago, when I w.
traught. I had no place to go, no way to turn, and I was ju
a mess. My husband went into these rages. I had no control of the finances, no money of my own, a low-paying
job, three children of high school age or lower, and the
worst downer for me was that there was no one who knew
what we were going through.

After a particularly frightening episode where my husband choked our seventeen-year-old daughter, I went to
the counseling center to try to get help for my daughter
and me. I was told at the center that if I said anything
about abuse to the counselor, or if my daughter did, this
would be reported to the authorities and my husband
would be taken to court, since my daughter was a minor.
The counselor further said that it does no good to bring
someone in and force them, via court order, to go to counseling. I was fearful for our lives if I pursued this, so we
both decided not to say anything about the abuse. We did
go on through a counseling program ourselves. My
daughter dropped out after a couple of sessions; I stayed
on for a year. My husband constantly badgered me about
going, saying that it was "costing us too much money." As
it turned out, everything was paid for through our health
insurance programs.

I lived in constant fear for my three daughters and
myself. Before we found the correct medication to help
with the violence, I had my neighbors alerted to the problems. They knew to let me in their door in the middle of
the night if I ran to their house in my night clothes. I had
a way to lock my bedroom door so that it would give me
time to get out the window if necessary. This was just a
nightmare period for me. The psychologist had me get rid
of John's gun. Fortunately, he has never noticed that it is
missing. We had this plan worked out that if he ques-

tioned me about it, I would say that another daughter and her husband had asked where it was, but I didn't know what had happened to it. But he has never asked. He is a perfect shot, by the way.

Even though things are better, I still have plans in place. If I call my daughter and tell her I will be over in ten minutes, she is to come over to our house if I do not show up. I stayed with her and her husband more than once.

Things smoothed off for awhile as the girls got older and went off to college. My husband knew that I was thinking very seriously about divorce, so that kept him from going into physical rages and beating us up. But things got progressively worse in other areas. He caused problems by scaring people at work and at meetings by going into rages there. Other symptoms appeared, and we finally realized that there was a big health issue here. In 1993, when physical symptoms appeared, we finally understood it was HD. The worst part for me during this time period was that I felt no one understood what the girls and I were going through, no one believed us, and we were on our own, in a sinking pool. The doctors sometimes give you the impression that you are making this up, as many have never had an HD patient. Plus, my husband always acted so normal when we went to the doctor.

After my arm was hurt and my husband told him there was nothing wrong with what he had done, the doctor put him on Mellaril. The doctor later told me that he wanted me to hear my husband's comments so I would understand how dangerous it was for me to live there.

My husband is on medication now. The girls are all grown up and gone, but the memories are still there. Our lives are a bit shattered, but we will make it. I have many regrets about what we went through and what I did and didn't do for the girls. It is very painful. Now we are in a "calm" phase due to the great medicines that are available. I have to keep up on everything that is happening just to stay ahead of things and not get caught again. I make sure he takes his pills. I keep the money that he gets in very small amounts so that he does not spend it on gin or scotch. I watch out for danger signals in his behavior and keep the doctors informed as to how he is doing on the current medications. When he seems unhappy, the first thing I do is unlock the door, and sometimes leave it ajar, to make sure I have an escape route. The way we are handling this keeps him at home, but I never relax my guard.

I don't have answers for anyone going through a situation like mine. But if you are scared, it is valid. Get some help for yourself. I still check in with a wonderful psychologist regularly. It helps me realize that I am OK and I can handle this. If possible, make sure that all of the professionals that are consulted really understand HD and what you are up against. I should have been more aggressive and reported the abuse even if it meant having the child protective services keeping guard over my children. It was not my fault and maybe had I reported the abuses, my husband would have been diagnosed more quickly and gotten the help he needed. I didn't do that for my children, and I regret that I didn't. Don't have the same regrets.

Protection At All Costs

My husband is in the hospital for the first time getting his medications balanced out. Under supervision, he can start new medication immediately, rather than wait the two and a half weeks to get the current medication completely out of his system. It is important to know how and when to switch drugs and what to use in dealing with the behavioral aspects of Huntington's Disease.

In the process of changing medications, my husband had a series of explosive outbursts that culminated in his pinning our eleven-year-old against a wall with his hand over his mouth and nose "in order to shut him up." The episode lasted all of ten seconds and there was no blood or bruises, but it scared the tar out of my poor kid. My husband then left, at his therapist's over-the-phone suggestion, and spent the night in a private park. He came back Wednesday morning and picked a verbal fight with our oldest, who is sixteen. When I offered solutions like staying with his stepdad, with church friends, or going to a hospital until the medication switch was complete, he demanded money and said he was going to leave me and file for divorce, and that I would never see him again. Not exactly sympathetic, I wrote him a large check, which my mom agreed to cover, and left to take the kids to school.

When I got back, he was on his knees praying, with tears running down his face. It was as if something disconnected had suddenly snapped back into place. He told me that God told him he owed his family whatever it took to keep all of us safe.

On Monday, we had talked to our family doctor about the increasing explosiveness, and his solution was to tell us he was looking for a new doctor for us. I think the copy of "A Physician's Guide to Huntington's Disease" I gave him scared him half to death! Fortunately, I found the phone number of a psychiatrist I had talked to in the past. Although she has little hands-on experience with HD, she seemed really knowledgeable.

I reached her Wednesday morning, and she talked to my husband and he agreed to check into the hospital, even though he has a terrible fear of never being let back out. Here they will work on stabilizing his medications.

I know I did the right things. I intervened between my husband and my kid. I told my kid to talk to the school counselor; it's a new school. I have discussed HD with the other two children and now we need to do it with this one too. I took my sick husband to the hospital to get him help. And what happens? I end up involved with Child Protective Services again. I don't get to talk to our prior caseworker, who had vindicated me when I explained HD and told her all the techniques we were using to cope. I have to start all over with a new person. Yes, I will probably be vindicated again; yes, they will still probably publicly pull my kids out of class to interview them separately "away from the home." And yes, they will probably leave a very public "urgent message from Child Protective Services" at my office. It's not good enough for them to talk to the school counselors and confirm that my kids haven't been physically harmed. It's not good enough to contact the kids' therapist and confirm that we are working on reassurance that it's "the disease, not the dad" and non-escalating coping skills. It's not good enough that a file already exists with all of the names and contact numbers of reliable, reputable people willing to say good things on behalf of the family, because they say, "That file is closed – each incident is handled separately."

Our state laws provide that doctors, hospitals, and schools must report any incident that involves physical contact with a child. It's enough to drive me back into the closet, swear my kids to secrecy, tell them not to talk to anybody except our private therapist, and drive to Mexico to get my husband's medications over-the-counter after, of course, quickly obtaining my degree in pharmacology, so I don't mis-prescribe. Actually, I'm just kidding. The secrecy isn't worth it at any price.

The issues surrounding Huntington's Disease are so varied that sometimes it is difficult to know where to start. HD has hurt so many people in so many ways. Of course my husband is suffering. He doesn't understand or like what is happening to him. But we don't either. The incidents of abuse and unacceptable behavior will only escalate if we don't take care of it now. I know it is the disease and not my husband, but it still a very real, very dangerous situation.

I hurt for my husband. I hurt for my children. I hurt for myself. But we are a family and I will do all in my power to protect everyone I love. If that means medication adjustments, counselors, psychiatrists, and even Child Protective Services, then so be it. It is worth it to protect those I love.

∽

Our Stories

BY ALBERT J. CERVI

It's interesting how one disease can be so different in two members of the same family. In 1966, after nineteen years of marriage, my wife began showing symptoms of Huntington's Disease, known back then as Huntington's Chorea. Bob, our only child, was sixteen years old.

My wife was not doing her housework right, her cooking was getting really bad, and she couldn't wash clothes anymore. One day, I noticed that when she sat down, she crossed her legs from right to left, then from left to right and back and forth incessantly. Her speech was getting blurred, one hand bent inwards towards her stomach, and at times she had a glassy stare. With effort, I could still understand what she was saying, but it was difficult. Though she had always had a good appetite, she stopped eating much and got weaker.

We liked to walk. I often held her under her good arm when we went the four blocks to my mother's house, and with her glassy eyes and her weak legs, people said she was drunk.

I took her to see the same doctor who had treated my mother-in-law who had died in 1933, at the age of forty-one, when the disease was called St. Vitus Dance. The doctor examined her and said, "Al, if she has what I think she does, I feel sorry for you." To be sure of his diagnosis, he sent us to Pittsburgh University where, after a complete examination, we were told that my wife did have this horrible disease. He told me what he knew of HD, and that I would have to place my wife in a hospital one day. I didn't do that right away; she did pretty well on her medicine for a time. But eventually, it became too much for me, and she went into the state hospital.

The first ten days of her stay, I was told not to visit or call. She would write letters to me, and when we finally got to come for visits, I would bring some of her favorite food and take her to the picnic grounds.

I took her home for weekends and holiday visits, and she did pretty good for a while. One Christmas, when she was home with us, she even walked the four blocks to my mother's house. I worked different times at the mill, so my mother was taking care of our son. After that short visit, she went back to the hospital and never walked again. I tried to find out why, but was never told what happened. Then on the next visit, they told me not to bring any more food or drinks because she was having trouble keeping anything down.

She continued to get worse and grew weaker, and during the last years in the hospital she never got out of bed. One night, in 1971, at the age of forty-six, she choked on some food and died. She'd been in the hospital for six years. Before she got sick, my wife was always a calm, quiet person; with Huntington's, she became very, very nervous, but not out of hand.

My son knew his mother had Huntington's, so when he joined the air force, he told them about his mother and they checked him for HD. When they told Bob he didn't have it, but that he should also never have children, he told his girlfriend about HD, and suggested they get married and just not have children. So they married and later adopted a little girl. It was better not to have children, just in case.

They moved down to Texas and then settled in California where he was transferred. First it was the car wrecks, some of them pretty bad, but he still kept driving. Later, Bob started to call me at all hours of the night, telling me he was seeing things that weren't there. Finally, after ten years of marriage, his wife divorced him.

In 1988, I got a medical flight to California where he was living by himself in very bad shape. Bob was pale and very thin, his tongue was swollen, his lips cracked and dry. I cleaned his house, made him meals, and got him ready to leave California. At first, Bob refused to go; for three days we talked and talked. Bob insisted he couldn't make the trip because his legs hurt and he wanted to go see his doctor. What he really wanted was for the doctor to say he couldn't travel. Of course, that was not an option as he could no longer take care of himself. He finally agreed that if we took his dog he would come back to Pennsylvania.

For a while, Bob ate more, watched TV, and generally did much better once he was home with me. Then one day, he faced the wall and started to repeat the Hail Mary over and over. I didn't say anything, just listened to him while my heart broke a little more. One night while in bed, Bob said, "I love you." I turned my head so he could not see me crying because I knew his downward spiral was continuing.

HD was taking my son, little by little. His mother had experienced mainly physical symptoms, but she stayed sweet and calm. Yes, she was nervous, but none of what had happened to her prepared me for Bob's behavior. One day, he shoved furniture up against the bedroom door so I couldn't open it. I was afraid he would go out the window, so I took the door off the hinges.

Bob was seeing two different doctors and was on medication, but when I gave him his pills, he would only pretend to take them and then put them in his pant's pocket. When I washed his clothes, I would find the pills. By early 1989, I had to take him to the local hospital; he was not eating or listening to me. He kicked the furniture and refused to do anything, no matter how I asked. After being in the hospital for a week, the doctors sent him home with a different medication.

Maybe it was all the stress of caring for Bob, but in February 1989, I had a heart attack. Thank goodness Bob was able to call for help even through his tears. I took care of Bob for a brief time after I was released from the hospital, but eventually, he went back to the hospital and then to a nursing home. After just a short time, he couldn't be controlled and I had to move him to a different nursing home. There, he continually swore at the help, refused to eat, and then one day he got out of the home. No one can say how it happened, but they found him on a main highway lying on the ground waiting to be hit by a truck. Because of this, he was moved to another hospital while arrangements were made to place him in the VA hospital.

Once, before he was admitted to the VA, he came home and his eight-year-old daughter came to visit. She flew all by herself from California and of course did not understand the sickness and why her daddy was as he was. One day she said, "I came all the way to see you and you won't even play ball with me." Oh, how he tried to play ball with his daughter – but he couldn't hold the bat. It was so sad to see the expectations of my granddaughter that would never be met.

In the middle of 1990, Bob finally entered the VA hospital. For over a year and a half, he refused to see me; he told the doctors I didn't want him. While there, he escaped and was found in the parking lot; this time, he said, waiting to get run over by a car. After that he was always strapped into a bed or a chair.

One day, he got quite ill from some sort of infection and asked to see me. After that, I would visit him weekly; sometimes two times and some of my family would come too. Bob never walked again after the infection. Not because he couldn't, but because he was tied down. No one ever walked him or tried to see what would happen if he was free. For five of his six years in this last hospital he never walked.

I would bring him the fruit pies he enjoyed and cream puffs; whatever Bob asked for, I would bring. Bob had stayed with my mother when my wife got sick, and in 1995, though she was ninety-eight years old, my mother would come with me to visit him. The doctors said we shouldn't keep anything from Bob and when my mother got sick and died, my sister told him. He cried for a while, but settled down during our visit.

One day, in July 1996, Bob beat himself up quite badly; they told me he banged himself against the bed repeatedly. The hospital called and suggested I not visit that day because of the his appearance. When I did see him, his head was cut, he was black and blue and his eyes were swollen. They placed his mattress inside an inflatable swimming pool so he could not hurt himself again.

In September, the hospital called, requesting we meet about Bob. My sister, her husband and I went to the meeting. They explained that Bob was slowly dying and there was nothing they could do; he might make it until Thanksgiving, surely not Christmas.

I spent as much time as possible with my son, and though he was dying, he still knew all of us. He had to be fed with a syringe by mouth because they did not want him to choke on food. On November 8, 1996, he seemed just as normal as on recent visits. As I was leaving, I said, "I'll see you on Sunday." He said, "Okay. Good-bye. So long." On the way home, I told my sister that Bob had said "so long" instead of "good-bye." That was odd for him and it worried me.

On Sunday, the roads were icy, so I called the hospital to see how Bob was doing. They told me he was eating and drinking, so I decided to wait and see him on Monday. But since the roads were unsafe again, I decided to wait. On Monday night at 10:55, the VA called to tell me Bob had passed away. A nurse had found him on her rounds. Bob's suffering was finally over.

Huntington's Disease is such a terrible disease for the person suffering and for those who love them. Like so many others, my wife never knew she was at-risk for HD. I heard about this book being written and wanted our stories told. I wanted to be able to let others know they are not alone in their suffering. I hope that someday soon there will be a cure, but in the meantime, I tell people to have courage and to know God is watching over them.

My Family, My Life

BY JIM GILES

Family is everything to me. My dad was a violent alcoholic and I think that influences how I feel about my current family. My older sister and I are very, very close. We always have been, and I think we always will be. Nita and I have been married for twenty-seven years; she was a little girl when we married and was still a little girl thirty years later. She always looked young and she got into places for child's prices when she was 34 years old. I am five years older then her and we have been mistaken for father and daughter many times.

We travelled around the world during my military career and Nita and my daughter, Jenny, made that very enjoyable. During those travels, we met many people who treated us as family and visa versa. Like other institutions, the military is just one big family. We now have friends that feel like family all over. Some of these people are as close as our blood family.

Nita miscarried while I was in Vietnam and again when we went to the Philippines. We went to Montana, and on a trip back home from California, we got caught in a snow storm in Cheyenne, WY and she miscarried there. Then Jenny was born, and two years later she miscarried again, so Jenny is very special to us.

Nita and I have had some very good years together. We have experienced the hardships and the joys of being in the military together and travelling the world. We were Girl Scout leaders and watched many girls become young ladies, along with Jenny. We did a large amount of traveling, camping and enjoying each other, and I would not change anything about that part of our lives. I guess you could say that I would be hollow, empty and unloved without my family. Love kept us going through some tough times in our lives and I expect it will continue to get us through.

Of course, there is a down side and that is the effects of HD on Jenny and Nita's relationship, especially when Jenny was a teen. Nita had moods, even before we knew it was HD. She tended to blame Jenny for many things that were imaginary, and as a result, they are were not as close as they might have been, when Jenny needed her most. The anger and rage that Nita has exhibited on a few occasions because of the HD is a very bad thing. We know it is the disease, but it is very hard for us not to take her verbal and physical attacks personally. But we do recover and accept it as a behavior of the disease and not a personal attack against us. Jenny has finally accepted this and they are much closer today.

Another sadness is that we had always planned to travel the country and visit all our friends that we made during our military years. Now, of course, HD is going to keep us from that dream.

I am often asked if I would have kids again if I knew about HD. My response is always the same. In a heartbeat. Jenny has provided so much joy for me that it is hard to imagine never having experienced that. As I said before, I would be hollow, empty and unloved without the experience of watching her become, grow and evolve. Nita is my love and my friend... Jenny is my life.

If I am a "good" daddy and a "great" granddad, it is out of love. My girls mean more to me than life itself. We have such a good time. Jenny and I used to have our own time together when she was little and I enjoyed her immensely. I still get tears in my eyes when I think about all we did together. Not the big things, but the little ones like going to a field and swinging her around and around, then chasing her and listening to her squeal. Carrying her around on my shoulders so she could see the world was a real treat for both of us. And having her run into my arms and give me a hug that stopped my breath could make my day. Watching her explore and find things out, teaching her about science and animals has helped to make her into the woman she is today. She has no fear of snakes and creepy crawly things, except spiders, and she loves the outdoors, the mountains, the desert and all animals. I like to think that I had a big influence in that part of her.

Now I get to do it all again with my granddaughter, Becca. She helps me in the garden and loves to play with worms, roly pollies, and snails. We have not caught a snake yet but we will someday, and she will grow up respecting them but not fearing them. She likes lizards, so snakes will be no problem. Becca loves me to swing her and carry her on my shoulders, going for walks, and she also is a great hugger and breath stealer; just like her mom. I love every minute of it. I am so glad I had a daughter and now a granddaughter; boys just would not have been the same for me.

Jenny recently married the son I never had. Indulge me if you will by allowing me to share a poem I wrote on that day.

My Daughter
BY JIM GILES

Twenty-three years ago
Almost to the day
You came into this world
In a very noisy way.

Your lips were all purple
Your skin was all pink
You were so special
Was all I could think.

The owies I've kissed
With love that did heal
The measles, the Pox
The sickness ordeals.

I can still remember
As you reached up to me
Screaming, "Swing me, Daddy, swing me."
As you giggled with glee.

I can still remember
The first time I heard
"Daddy, I love you.
Do you love me too?"

I traveled the world
With your mother and you
You took England by storm
The only "Yank" in their school.

FACES OF HUNTINGTON'S

We had a great time there
We two, plus you.
The visits to Birdland
And the Cotswolds too.

We returned to the States
To begin a new phase
You had grown into a young lady
But you still were my 'babe.'

You made it through grade school
With much pomp and circumstance
And on to the middle school
You were always advanced.

Then came those early teen years
They were so hard on you
"No, Baby, because I love you
Do you still love me too?"

Then you got your driver's license
And my whole world changed
You had your freedom
I had to release the reins.

You were my little girl
I love you so dear
I wanted to protect you
And keep you so near.

Now you are no little girl
You are a woman today
It's time to turn you loose
It's time to give you away.

My little girl
You will forever be
And I hope to always hear
Those words so dear to me.

"Daddy, I love you
Do you love me too?"

The Father of the Bride, April 12, 1997

~ 9

Christine's Story

BY CHRISTINE PATERNOSTER

I CAN scarcely remember the years gone by when I first heard the words "Huntington's Disease." Little did I know that it would change my entire life, and not entirely for the worse as one might think.

I guess my earliest memory of dating my husband, John, is that I was so comfortable with him. It was sort of like having a best friend and older brother all wrapped into one. It wasn't love at first sight, but rather a gradual warming that developed into a deep and committed love between us. Maybe that is why we made it through extremely difficult years.

John was always nervous and fidgety. As the years passed, HD was presenting itself, but we were not aware of its subtle and sneaky entrance into our lives. Gradually, John deteriorated to the point where he fell a great deal, was easily confused, could never finish a project, and slurred words. He went to a neurologist for frequent and severe headaches and was diagnosed with a movement disorder called Tourette's Syndrome.

Every time someone who had not seen him in a while asked me what was wrong, I would always answer, "The doctor says he has a movement disorder but it's nothing serious; we learn to live with it." As time went on, he worsened, but the doctors had me convinced I was over-reacting. Finally, in 1986, his company forced him onto disability and early retirement because he kept falling at work and was forgetful in his responsibilities.

At this point, his father pulled me aside and told me John had been adopted. Before John's adopted mother died when he was thirteen, his father had promised he would never tell John about the adoption. I was angry not only for John, but for myself. When you marry someone, you assume his parents are as presented. Upon hearing the news, we never considered a genetic disease. Instead, I was upset because I didn't know what nationality my children really were. Coming from a first generation German heritage, this was important to me. I was soon to learn how irrelevant that was and that it was the least of my worries.

After the news, a friend of the family asked if John had ever been tested for HD. I didn't even know what it was, but went to the library and found a small paragraph about the disorder. Brief as it was, it was enough for me to know what had been going wrong all these years. I found a new neurologist and advised him of my concerns. Even with the lack of family history, John received a diagnosis on his first visit, though I didn't tell John right away. I've learned in life that these things are best not planned, and circumstances will present themselves in the future to allow the truth to emerge.

Life went on and we all adjusted. By the time of his diagnosis, we had three daughters, and in spite of his illness, we were happy. Although not working, he could do simple chores around the house, get the kids off to school, and be there for them when they got home. I continued to work outside the home taking over the role of bread winner. By 1989 and 1990, he had reached the point where he was having difficulty swallowing, couldn't shower, shave or dress himself. I knew that home health care would be needed to assist in his daily care while I was at work.

My middle daughter, Jamie, age twelve at the time, began having seizures. She had always had speech problems and frequently stuttered, but by this time, she tested low enough for special education classes. I still had not considered Huntington's as a possibility since I considered myself well read on the subject, and juvenile HD was supposedly rare.

By the end of 1990, John couldn't swallow, was constantly choking and had lost forty pounds. The doctors suggested a feeding tube so that is what we did. We did not realize we had a choice. On Christmas Eve, he left the hospital and I continued to take care of him at home.

The strain of caring for him, parenting three children and working became increasingly difficult. Dementia appeared with a vengeance, wreaking havoc and producing violent temper tantrums. The alarm awoke everyone in the house as he climbed over the side of the hospital bed all night long, dragging the feeding pump with him. With all that was going on, I was of no use to anyone. It became obvious that a nursing home was needed so that I could care for my children and myself, and still hold down a job.

Jamie, by now thirteen years old, was diagnosed with HD. On the heels of the diagnosis, Jennifer, my youngest at age nine, began showing some fidgety movements. She was already in speech and special education, following Jamie's path. I knew in my heart that HD had claimed another victim, but could only handle the crisis I was facing with John and Jamie at the time. I refused to consider that Jennifer had it too. During the summer of 1991, I took the children on a long weekend to an out-of-state amusement park where Jennifer had a seizure. While the paramedics kept assuring me that seizures are common in children and can be the result of many causes, the incident was the confirmation I needed; Jennifer was following in her sister's footsteps.

John went into a nursing home in February, got pneumonia in August, and died on September 10, 1991. I felt an immediate sense of tremendous loss but also an inner peace. My daughters each took his death in her own way, and I was pleased that we had so many happy memories. While I had felt like a single parent and had the full responsibility of the house and children long before John died, grief is still a long and necessary road we all must follow. Taking a shortcut or going over or around it only prolongs the process.

A few months after John died, I noticed my sixteen-year-old daughter Kim making some awkward movements. I chalked that up to being a clumsy teenager along with the slurred speech being because of her braces. She was having difficulty keeping up with her classes academically, but I reasoned, "OK, she's not a genius, but I can live with that." Then one day, she displayed a typical HD movement, and I knew she had it too. However, in my customary style, I tucked it away until I could deal with it since there was nothing to be done at that point anyway.

As the months passed, however, Kim began exhibiting aggressive behavior at home with her sisters and myself. The explosiveness became violence and I finally reached a point where I realized she would need to be on medication, and I would need a diagnosis to justify the treatment.

She was diagnosed, referred to a psychiatrist, then began taking an anti-anxiety medication and going to counseling two or three times a month. Most times, home life was tolerable, but that's just it... barely tolerable. At times, in my day to day life, I was hanging by a thread. Most nursing homes won't take one HD patient. Can you imagine living with three?

I gave up asking, "Why me? Why all three? Why was I picked to carry this burden?" I don't know and I don't think I'll ever know. HD, like any other disease or crisis in life, has its benefits. Looking back, I wouldn't change a thing. My faith has deepened and when I ask God for strength, I get it. "Why" doesn't matter anymore. I have a wonderful family and friends who are a great support. When I realized I would only have my children for a short time, I tried to make their lives the best I could and I tried to cherish them in every way possible. I also forgave myself for losing patience and forced myself to get away from time to time. I'm blessed with a wonderful employer and truly caring, compassionate friends, some of whom face HD in themselves or families, but many more that don't.

On April 10, 1995, Jamie died at the age of sixteen, with Jennifer taking her last breath on May 17, 1997. I am now the caregiver of my oldest daughter, Kimberly, who is twenty and confined to a wheelchair with slurred speech and still difficult, but tolerable, behavior. Her smile and giggles are my reward.

Yes, I do feel cheated. But I couldn't be more proud of my daughters than if they had won the Nobel Prize, because they are the most courageous of heroes. So many people, teachers, doctors, nurses, and aides have told me what a joy my children are and what an inspiration I am. Maybe this is what God's plan was for me. He gave me strength so that I could help others. All I know is that I am not the same person I was before all this happened to me, and my life has become richer and more fulfilling because of these experiences. I hope that someday you will be able to look back at your life and say the same.

10

Faces of Heroes

BY CARMEN LEAL-POCK

*L*ife shrinks or expands in proportion to one's courage.

—Anais Nin

In mythology, heroes are often of divine ancestry. They are endowed with great courage and strength, celebrated for bold exploits, and favored by the gods. Legendary heroes can be persons noted for feats of valor, or nobility of purpose, especially those who have risked or sacrificed life or limb. Victims and caregivers of Huntington's Disease do not belong to mythology, because mythical heroes are fictional. But they are legendary, because they are heroes of supreme courage and strength.

Heroes come in many shapes and sizes and from all economic and racial backgrounds. There are those who have fought in wars to ensure freedoms. Doctors continue to help solve medical mysteries, while sports heroes give us enjoyment as we cheer them on. From businessmen to inventors to movie stars, when asked, we can all ramble off the names of our heroes. Amazingly enough, some of our heroes are even politicians.

To me, the real heroes in this world are usually those who live their lives in a way dedicated to helping others. Arthur Ashe said, "True heroism is remarkably sober, very undramatic. It is not the urge to surpass all others at whatever cost, but the urge to serve others whatever the cost." When I think of that definition, I recall many names of heroes that have gone unnoticed. It has been said that heroism consists of hanging on one minute longer. In both definitions of heroism, I know individuals who are fighting the beast called Huntington's Disease.

A person with HD continuing to function, against all odds, within his or her family and community, is a hero. When I hear of a caregiver who works full time, raises kids and gives care to a loved one with HD, I know there walks a hero. Members of the medical and research professions that make strides in caring for and curing HD are truly heroes in this battle. Who can question the heroism of those who give compassionate care to those in need?

I find that, in reality, the majority of heros I know have names that are unrecognizable to most of the world. They are simply doing their jobs in the best way they know how.

One of these heroes is a home health nurse for two brothers who have HD. Ken and Gary are still able to live on their own in a small trailer in the back of their mother's house. It is an ideal arrangement for helping them remain independent. Without the help of their nurse, however, they quite possibly would not be able to stay alone.

Ken and Gary's mom, Shirley, can't praise Veronica enough.

"She is a heroine in our lives because of being so special," says Shirley. "Ken and Gary do not have a lot to say, but she (Veronica) can somehow get them to communicate.

She brings special little treats, but then again, she does this for all her patients. Veronica copies anything that she sees on HD and brings it to me, reads all the information I give her, and is very persistent with our neurologist. Ken and Gary both love children dearly and she has brought her young son and daughter to visit them. She is a very special person as she does little favors for all of her patients, usually spending her own money for the treats and for gas." Shirley continues, "We are the main priority on her prayer list at church, and she has offered to stay with the guys while Jerry and I go to church or out to eat. I have never met anyone more caring, and feel that we are blessed to have her assigned to us."

Jeanette has also been blessed by having an exceptional home health aide to care for her son. This is what she has to say about the care her son, Ken, is receiving. "Over the last couple of years, we have had several aides that come to help Ken with his bathing and other personal grooming. There are very few people in the health profession that understand what Huntington's families go through. After finally being approved for home health care, I was sent a wonderful aide. Not only is she (Vicki) a dedicated worker, but she is part of an HD family. She had a twin brother who died of Huntington's, cancer and AIDS. Vicki is now taking care of a second brother that has HD. She is working on the possibility of removing a third brother from the home where he is presently, and caring for him as well. A goal of hers is to run a daycare center or a home for those with Huntington's Disease."

Taking care of a beloved member of your family with Huntington's Disease is tough. But to plan on taking care of more than one is heroic.

Trisha tells about a couple in her church who were heroes at a time when her father-in-law needed to be rescued. "My father-in-law, Tom, was placed in the Veteran's Administration hospital when my mother-in-law could no longer care for him on her own. Charlotte had little money, less federal assistance, and with no one to help, was virtually on her own. She attends a church that, at the time, had a temporary pastor. Pastor Bob and his wife served at the church for less than a year, until a permanent replacement came. After he spent some time in the Dedham, Massachusetts Veteran's Administration hospital, the VA wanted to transfer Tom to Maine. Dedham was conveniently located only twenty minutes away, while Maine is a drive of several hours. Pastor Bob's wife, Estelle, had a brother who worked for the VA in Albany, NY, who requested that Tom be transferred to Albany as his patient. After six months there, Tom could be relocated to a facility closer to home."

"Pastor Bob and Estelle had relocated to Albany," Trisha goes on, "and when Charlotte and my husband traveled to Albany every other weekend to see Tom, they were able to stay with them. What a blessing they were. During these weekend visits, Tom could leave the hospital because of these lovely people, and they were able to feed him, do his laundry, and care for him. House guests can get old quickly, yet these caring people opened their home every other weekend for six months. Something even more amazing is that on the alternating weekends, they themselves would take him out of the hospital and provide the same loving care for Tom. They were no longer at the same church attended by my mother-in-law, yet they cared enough to make sure Tom was not alone. They are unsung heroes who continue to touch my life."

Another hero is Bobby Basco. Mary's daughter, Annette, has HD, inherited from her father. Bobby was married to Annette's aunt, who so far has no HD symptoms. Bobby is an ordinary guy. When Annette was five or six, Bobby and his wife divorced. Every so often they exchanged an occasional phone call, but that was the extent of the relationship.

"When Ryan, Annette's dad, became symptomatic," Mary shares, "Bob began to help us in many ways. I remember his bringing Ryan to the local mental health facility at 2:00 a.m. so that he could be evaluated by a neurologist from New Orleans, who worked pro bono for the hospital. Of course, since he was working for free, he worked odd hours. It was cold and dark. I was afraid, and Ryan was big and strong and increasingly aggressive. I was frightened of him, but I knew I had to keep the appointment. Though he was not on a white horse, Bobby was my hero nonetheless. He arrived with Ryan in tow, calm and smiling.

"Bobby walked with me through the horrendous Social Security process. He also provided Ryan with a place to live, a pseudo-family, food, outings, and a safe place for me to bring Annette to see her dad. He cut his hair, shaved his face, and talked to him when everyone else considered him dead. After Ryan had to go to a nursing home, Bobby and his new wife went everyday to feed him, see that he was comfortable, and ensure that his needs were met. They certainly didn't care for him out of duty or kinship since they were not kin. Nor were they there for him out of any sort of obligation. Bobby just did it for him until Ryan died, and then he helped me to bury him properly, and paid for the funeral. I guess it was him, because I know I did not pay the bill."

One of the joys in creating this book has been in sorting through the stories that come my way from people who are in some way involved with Huntington's Disease. I could, and probably should, write an entire book focusing on the unsung heroes that help in ways both large and small. One of those heroes came into my life through an E-mail message this morning. This is what he said:

"As a physician, I had a walnut wall covered with plaques. I stripped that wall, because none of the awards were given to me for things I did that were at great personal expense to me and sometimes my family.

"I have sent this to you privately, because I have my own agedness and medical problem, which would prevent me from responding to even a small number of E-mails, but I wanted you to see it and cheer you on with what you are doing. By the way, I have treated close to three hundred pHD's. They were my special patients. Though their lives were often robbed from them and their families, and there was much agony endured by all, they have often, in our endeavors to care for them, brought out the best qualities in us as human beings."

This physician is a hero not only for his compassion and no doubt excellent care he has given his patients, but for understanding that often it is those with the least to give that give the most. What followed was a remarkable poem from a most remarkable man. He chooses to remain anonymous, though he did give permission for me to use the poem, which is very personal to him.

The Walnut Wall

The wall of walnut is bare now.
It was the bearer of awards and honors.
Now it bears but beams and beams
at our folly as it bares the truth
that honors are not worthy of the walnut
upon which they hang nor represent deeds of quiet honor.
The splashy plaquered wall misdirected us
to obvious deeds... often misdeeds of pride and selfish ambitions...
a Noblest Prize not nobly won.
The sole, soul-directing deed was
the stripping of the wall of its plaquered veneer.

Sit quietly, my friend, at the base of the stripped wall
in a state of one stripped soul,
not at all bare, but richly reflecting
quiet kindnesses of those
whose kindness is heralded by unheraldedness,
and whose splashiness is the absence of splash
and whose deeds were indeed free gifts without recorded deed.

There are other heroes I have not met in person. The on-line support group is filled with heroes. When I asked the list to suggest who were the heroes in their lives, two names were mentioned by Ginny.

The first name was Jean Miller. Jean is Kelly's mother and Kelly has juvenile HD. Ginny's daughter, Pam, has juvenile HD, too. Unless you have been a parent of a terminally ill child, I imagine it is hard to find someone to relate to about your situation. "Jean came into my life when I was alone in my fight against HD. She inspired me to look the beast in its eyes and fight to destroy it. Through the Internet, Jean has brought moral support and knowledge to people around the world at the first call for help. She is always there even though she herself must fight against her beautiful daughter being trampled by the beast. She reaps no publicity, no rewards for her efforts but her own inner satisfaction. Jean Miller is truly one of life's true heroes."

Daria and her husband had no idea that HD loomed in their future, since he was adopted. When they learned of his at-risk status, they were frightened and confused. "Though the years of respite from HD were peaceful in retrospect, the wake-up call, when it came, was horrible in the worst sense of the word. I am forever grateful that the first person who responded to our pitiful cry for help was Jean Miller. She was a hand reaching out, beyond the worst day imaginable, to pull us back into the world of the living; a single candle lit in a horrible darkness. She let us know that we would survive and things hopefully would be all right. Without her, I don't know. Jean led us to this list. Perhaps we would have achieved the peace we have thus far, but I tend to doubt it. Knowledge is power, and she gave us our first taste of knowledge concerning HD. For this, I will be forever grateful to Jean."

Another hero mentioned by several is a man by the name of Jim Pollard. Jim is the administrator of a nursing home in Lowell, Massachusetts. They care for one of the largest concentrated groups of pHD's in the nation. As Ginny puts it, "Jim Pollard has dedicated so much of his life to help families with HD. Jim is fortunate enough to have a family that is untouched by HD, yet he strives to help us all. Jim could enter the world of HD at 8:00 a.m. and leave it at 4:00 p.m. He could go to a few required meetings with staff and family and that could be the extent of his HD involvement. Instead, our Jim has dedicated himself unselfishly to find new ways to make people with HD comfortable and independent. He has brought support and imaginative ideas to the entire HD community."

The world is filled with heroes; from those whose names are famous throughout the world, to those ordinary people just living their lives the way they have been taught. Both types of heroes give us hope and help us through rough periods. I am thankful for the heroes of Huntington's.

∽

The Kites

BY CARMEN LEAL-POCK

"True courage is like a kite; a contrary wind raises it higher."

—John Petit-Senn

The kite danced upwards. Its turquoise color blended with the ocean fronting the sandy beach. If you squinted, you could see the black and white applique shape of the killer whale on the turquoise background as it rocketed to and fro. The little boy's face, as he flew his kite, was wreathed in a smile even brighter than the sun.

In sharp contrast to this happy child was a second boy, with a dejected slump to his shoulders. His kite was lying on the grassy field, looking even more forlorn than its owner. He was an ambitious boy, determined to fly the more complicated "trick" kite. Unlike the simplistic toy used by his brother, this kite had two strings and required either extensive experience, or a second pair of hands.

As I watched, I focused on the second boy who tenaciously pursued his work of getting the kite to fly. Each time he tried, he inched farther down the road to success.

And with each success, the kite whirled and danced in a way that showed how much more exciting and intricate the dance would be when the kite finally took flight. Each time it looked as though the boy would give up, I saw a squaring of his shoulders. Conviction on his face told me he would succeed if he had to stay up all night.

As the day wore on, the appearance of the second boy's kite, faded by the sun to a worn, soft color, with its grass and dirt smudges from having repeatedly been dropped to the ground, began to seem familiar; it reminded me of my husband, David, and what his life was like.

Huntington's Disease makes Dave look faded and tired most days. Like the second kite, he has to have help to do so many things. The trick kite is best flown with two pairs of hands. It is possible with one, but it is a struggle. Dave used to use only one pair of hands when he was an athlete, a computer whiz and a builder of houses. Dave was a special man; a wonderful husband and friend.

Now it is hard for Dave to do most anything without a second pair of hands. He requires help with eating and bathing and dressing. Even walking is becoming difficult as his unsteady gait causes him to pitch forward. His slurred speech causes confusion. He requires medication to quiet his troubled mind.

I thought about how much David had lost of himself as I observed the bedraggled kite swirl and dance across the sky. It seemed as if it had taken on a life of its own. The second boy had managed to lift the kite, and the joy on his face was delightful.

Looking at the kite in the sky, I thought about the superhuman effort David exerted going to work each day before diagnosis. I remembered the times he dressed and fed himself when it didn't seem possible. Each time David had a personal victory, it was a tenacious feat. His simple, quiet dignity as he learned to ask for help was humbling to see. His pride in completing a task, alone or aided, reminded me of the little boy who had managed to bring the trick kite to life.

Dave is a man comfortable with who he is. He can find contentment in ways I never would have thought possible. The victories I take for granted and measure as small send Dave soaring as high as that trick kite. There will be more and greater struggles as this disease continues ravaging his brain. There will come a time when it appears the Dave I know and love is no longer flying, like that trick kite. I know, though, my Dave is always there, even if I can't see him.

Some people seem to be uncomplicated. Their lives are easy as the small triangle kite the first boy put to flight so effortlessly. Theirs are also lives that don't affect others as profoundly as Dave's. Dave has touched many people because of the dignity with which he is facing the inevitable. He has touched my life. He is truly soaring high with each breath he takes.

The next time I see a scrap of fabric dancing in the sky, taking unimaginable dives that defy explanation, I will think of David. I will also think of the many people with Huntington's Disease who are changing lives. They have immense courage and they are all heroes.

∽

Jim Sauer, PhD, pHD

BY MARY S. PRICE

Surely most families have someone like Jim; stories and legends are woven around people like him. Jim is one of my younger brothers. He had a way about him; some called him eccentric, others admired his sense of adventure, his independence and his relentless pursuit of all subjects that were of interest to him.

Jim was, and still is, an archaeologist. Somehow, that description does not quite do him justice. From the age of sixteen, ever since he accompanied my parents on a trip to the Middle East, he has lived and breathed archeology. For my dad, archaeology was an avocation. For Jim, it became a passionate and consuming vocation that took him from Boston, where he earned a PhD in archaeology, to various locations in the Middle East. There he often represented the American Society of Oriental Research (ASOR) in a variety of archaeological pursuits.

While on a dig in Jordan, he met a lovely American woman named Sue, and shortly thereafter they were married. They subsequently had two children: Katie, who writes beautiful poetry, and Tom, an ardent outdoorsman who excels at fishing. The four of them returned to the United States and eventually settled in the Boston area, where Jim was one of the curators at the Harvard Semitic Museum. After several months of mysterious symptoms, Huntington's Disease was first identified and diagnosed in our family. Jim's announcement generated the kind of shock, confusion, and turmoil that most families touched by HD experience.

Recognizing that several archaeological projects were still in progress, Jim quickly realized that they needed to be concluded sooner rather than later. The academic future that had appeared seemingly endless was suddenly being collapsed into a few short months. Jim had not only his professional dedication, but the loyal assistance of our Mum whose organizational skills, sense of humor and eternal optimism greatly contributed to the successful outcome of these efforts. Jim managed to complete most of the projects that required his unique skills and experience before the effects of HD became too much for that kind of work.

Perhaps the best recognition of Jim's professional contributions was captured in a report of an ASOR reception honoring him, published in *Biblical Archaeology Review* in April 1997. The report said, "...I cannot refrain from mentioning the emotional ASOR reception that honored its former, two-term, fifty-one-year-old president, James Sauer. Several years ago, Sauer contracted a fatal malady, Huntington's Disease, and had to give up his academic activities. Although obviously infirm, he was able to accept the tribute of his crowds of admirers and to respond graciously. From 1975 to 1981, Sauer headed the American Center of Oriental Research in Amman, revitalizing archaeology in Jordan. Prince Raad bin Seid, Lord Chamberlain to Jordan's King Hussein, flew in from Amman to present Sauer with the special award medal called the Order of the Star."*

Hearing and reading the reports of this recognition of Jim's professional contributions reminded me again of all that the rest of my family and I have learned from Jim on a more personal level. I marvel at his appreciation for the past (without trying to hold onto to it unduly). I am awed by his undiluted enthusiasm for the present moment, and his remarkable ability to focus decisively on whatever was immediately at hand that required his undivided attention. I have found hope in his never-ending hope for the future together with his abiding conviction that it will be worth waiting for and that it will be good. While that future is not what it once was for Jim, he is facing this part of his life's journey with the same sense of personal honesty, integrity and dignity that typified the rest of his life. Not even HD could take that from him or from us.

---

* "New Orleans Gumbo: Plenty of Spice at Annual Meeting" by Hershel Shanks. Volume 23, No. 2 (Mar/Apr 1997) p. 69.

My Dad, My Hero

BY SHANA MARTIN

Things began to change when I was in kindergarten. Until then, I was like most kids and had a happy home, with a father and mother who loved each other. I was an only child, but that was fine. Having such great parents more than made up for the lack of siblings.

My mother started acting differently when I was five, as if there was something wrong with her both mentally and physically. Her hands and feet would twitch and she forgot things very easily. She would also get mad very easily, which was hard for a five-year-old to understand.

Although my dad took her to many doctors, none of them could figure out what was wrong with my mom. Finally, we took her to the Mayo Clinic in Minnesota where we were told she had a degenerative brain disorder called Huntington's Disease. Besides being rare, it was also terminal; her mental and physical conditions would continue to worsen until the end.

Both of my parents were determined to make the best of it. My mother continued to get very sick, and she would get mad and throw fits. She had trouble swallowing, and as a result, it became harder and harder for her to eat. After that, the falling started. She wanted so badly to stay the same and unaffected by the disease; she constantly tried to do things that were beyond her lessening abilities. She would fall a lot, which resulted in her being taken to the hospital at least once a week.

One night, when I was in third grade, Mom brushed up against the stove in the kitchen. Her robe caught on fire and she screamed. My dad ran in and ripped off her burning clothes, and put out the fire. He saved her life, but burned his hands.

Those were tough years for all of us in different ways. Many caregivers put their loved ones in nursing homes as soon as any problem occurs. My dad refused to do this. We got to the point where Mom could not be left in the house alone because she was a constant danger to herself. Though I was very young, Dad and I would trade shifts taking care of her. Many times he would sit with her all night, just to make sure she was okay. When it finally came time for Mom to move into a nursing home, my dad had the hardest time dealing with it and went into a depression. Even with that, he managed to carry on with his day-to-day activities.

We now visit my mother at least once or twice a week. No matter how busy I am with school, my dad makes sure we go to see her and that we don't miss a scheduled visit. He also gives talks at the home so the nurses understand the disease better. If they ever need help caring for Mom, he is right there.

The other day, Dad taped a news magazine show on television and insisted I watch one of the segments. It was a meaningful story about a woman who was in a coma, and when she awoke, she was completely paralyzed. She had no way to communicate, but was well aware of all that was going on around her. People thought she was still in a coma. She heard herself referred to as, "The Vegetable," and couldn't let anyone know that was not true. Finally, even her family stopped visiting her. After seven years, a speech therapist realized that she was indeed not in a coma, only paralyzed. With her dedicated assistance, this woman was able to learn to communicate through blinking.

My dad wanted me to watch this show because of my mother. Mom is at the stage where she can no longer communicate. She is stiff in a wheelchair and must have someone to help her do everything, including feed her. Dad explained that Mom was like the lady in the story, and we must never allow her to be ignored or abandoned. We need to talk to her and tell her what is going on around her.

There were times when I wasn't able to believe this, when I didn't even think my mother knew who I was. But recently there have been several signs that she is not only aware of me, she delights in my presence. When I spoke to her about my prom, she turned her head and looked at me as if she desperately wanted to say something and I knew my dad was right. He is a very smart man.

Throughout all that we have been through with my mother, Dad still wants me to have the best life a girl could have. When I was very young, we travelled around the United States so I could learn about the history and different people of our country. When I was old enough to participate in sports, I was enrolled in swimming, ballet, and gymnastics. Since I was an only child, he wanted to make sure I had plenty of friends around me. He even got me a bunk bed for sleep-overs. He never wanted me to be lonely. During the summers he let me choose what camps to go to so I could learn new things. He let me join any sport that interested me, and I excelled in gymnastics and logrolling.

I now earn all my money from logrolling and am also a varsity gymnast, which has made me stronger both physically and mentally. I recently started karate, another sport at which I am excelling. When my mom could still travel, all three of us went to Egypt and Israel. Dad also takes me across the country to my tournaments and has introduced me to backpacking and other outdoor activities.

Sometimes, when a parent gets sick, the remaining parent chooses who needs the most attention. When that happens, somebody ends up feeling less important, and that hurts. My dad didn't stop caring for my mother or me when she became ill. He wanted both of us to have the best lives possible given the circumstances.

I do wish I had a mother to share things with like my friends. But I have seen my dad love my mother in a special way, and that has taught me many lessons. I know Dad loves me and wants all the best for me. My dad is the most special man I know. My dad is my hero.

∽

A Family of Heroes

BY DIANA FISHER

I first discovered there was Huntington's Disease in my family after I was engaged to be married. My father came to me and told me he didn't know much about this disease, but my grandfather had told him that it was in the family. It seems my cousin had committed suicide because he thought he was getting the symptoms; the sad fact is that he didn't have it when they did the autopsy. But the note he left indicated that he thought he did.

My parents, Robert and Marjorie, married after instant love and a four-month courtship. Blessed with three daughters, life was good. One night in 1971, my father was visiting his father-in-law when the conversation drifted to the funeral of the cousin who had committed suicide. It was then that my father first heard the words "Huntington's Chorea," and that it could have an impact on his world.

My father decided, since my mother never mentioned it, she must not want to talk about it. He told her he had just found out from her father that her mother, Lilly, had died of HD. It seems my grandmother was at her worst when my mom was away to college, so they didn't tell her for fear she would quit school and come home to take care of her. Lilly died in 1949 of pneumonia, following several choking incidents. My uncle knows the most about the tough times the family went through, but he avoids talking about it because it is still too painful.

Since my father didn't know much about the disease and I needed to explain it to my fiancé, I made an appointment with my doctor to get more information. We both went to see him in 1972. He said he didn't know much about it either, but he referred me to a Dr. Hans Zelleweger in Iowa City, who was doing research on genetic diseases. This doctor had heard about a family in Adair County, Iowa, that had Huntington's Disease, but, according to Dr. Zelleweger, the "hick doctor in Greenfield" wouldn't share any information.

I tried to get some information from the doctor in Greenfield, but I finally figured out he really didn't know much about the disease. In Adair County, it was known by many as "Bochart Craziness," because of the eight out of eleven children who died with this disease in the 1920s and 30s. My grandmother's name was Lilly Emma Kathryn Bochart ; and she was one of those Bocharts. And now there was another generation with it. I began working with Dr. Zelleweger on this project. I drew up a family tree for him and told relatives it was a project for college.

My father and I did not discuss this in front of my mother. We knew at least one of her brothers had HD, and we believed she didn't want to talk about it. Mom was a teacher. One night, when she had a meeting scheduled after school, Dad and I spread everything out on the table to put it together for Dr. Zelleweger. As we were working, she walked in the door. Our mouths dropped open when she walked in the door as we were working. There was no hiding what we were doing.

"What is going on here?" she asked. "Aren't we going to use the table to eat on?"

We explained that we thought she had a meeting. After she told us it had been canceled, Dad showed her what we were doing.

Expecting her to be angry with us, we were shocked by her reaction. She was in the dark, not even realizing her brother had HD; she had thought it was Multiple Sclerosis. Mom also had no idea that her mother had suffered with Huntington's Disease. She had been told her mother had developed problems after a car accident and the trauma affected her "that way." When questioned on the cause of her mother's death, the doctor had said, "Nothing for you to be concerned about."

There have been various accepted HD myths, and the doctor had shared this one with my mother. He held to the belief that HD was only passed from mothers to sons, of which she had three. Mom was the only daughter. Even so, I don't know why he thought she wouldn't be concerned; these were her brothers or cousins or nephews that could possibly get this terrible disease.

My father's mother began helping Mom find information about HD, and we sought out the Iowa Chapter of the Committee to Combat Huntington's Disease. They visited with Marjorie Guthrie and became very involved in trying to find a cure. In the course of learning more about HD, my mother went to a meeting were she heard Dr. Guessella and Dr. Conneally speak about the need for more families to get involved. Because HD is a genetic disease, it was important to find affected families for research purposes.

If you ever talk to Dr. Conneally, he will tell you this story a hundred times. My mother called and then wrote to Dr. Conneally trying to get him to use her family for research. He was in Indiana and she was in Iowa. Finally,

Dr. Conneally wrote her stating that if she could get ten family members together, he would consider working something out.

She called him and asked if he meant ten people or one hundred. He confirmed that he needed ten family members. She exclaimed that her family had one hundred members who would be interested in participating. That was all the convincing Dr. Conneally needed. He told her to set up a location, because he and his staff were coming to Iowa to do some research.

Our family first gathered at Grand View College in Des Moines. Doctors and others doing genetic research were there for our footprints, blood, urine, saliva, and even taste tests. It was, to put it mildly, a very strange family reunion. After the battery of tests, Dr. Conneally and his associates came back to a nursing home in Adair, Iowa. There they drew more blood and tissue to clone from a select few family members.

The conversations and research began in the late 1970s, and the marker for the gene was found in 1983, as well as the presymptomatic test for Huntington's Disease. They found it in the Iowa family and confirmed it with the Venezuela Collaborative Huntington's Disease Project. That landmark finding demonstrated for the first time that the newly developed DNA markers could be used successfully to map human genes.

Dr. Conneally was ecstatic at locating the gene, but there was also a sadness at the discovery. The women who had worked so hard to set this large family base up for them had the marker. Yes, my mother, Marjorie Helen Jensen, had the marker for Huntington's Disease. She didn't know it and she wasn't showing any signs, but it was there.

Dr. Conneally continued a close relationship with my mother as he did his follow-up study on the progress of this disease in my family. As he requested, she didn't write anything down, and he used numbers to protect confidentiality. He thought that project ended in May 1989, when she died of a blocked colon, not showing any predominate signs of HD.

At the 1989 HDSA Convention in San Francisco, Dr. Conneally tearfully revealed to my sister, Roberta, and me, that Mom had the marker for HD. This news meant we were still at-risk. We both attempted to pick up where Mom left off on the research, assisting Dr. Conneally anytime we could. We also heard at that convention that HD research had just received a brain from someone who had died a few months before the convention. The donor had the marker, was non-symptomatic, and died of something totally unrelated. Why was that so important? This brain had narrowed the road to the gene. Researchers said it was "like narrowing a five hundred mile road down to one hundred miles." They were getting closer. My sister and I believe that brain was my mother's. It may not have been, but it does make dealing with her death more bearable.

Then in 1993, they found it. The Gene. We were able to test my mother's blood for the Huntington's gene at Indiana University where her blood is banked. Before that, my sister and I were both tested. Mom's CAG numbers were forty-two and seventeen. Both my sister and I have seventeen and nineteen. We don't know what my middle sister's numbers are, since she doesn't choose to know yet.

Taking the gene test is the hardest test in the world I have ever taken; and I am a teacher, certified medication aide, emergency medical tech, and professional photographer. I have had a few tests in my day, and this is one where I was thrilled to receive a negative result.

Our family received the Milton Wexler Foundation Award at the National HDSA Convention held in Des

Moines, Iowa in 1991. As president of the Iowa Chapter, I had been conducting the meetings and had no idea this was going to happen. When Nancy Wexler, one of the researchers working with Dr. Conneally, handed my father and I this beautiful large plaque, I was utterly speechless. My father still has it wrapped in a bath towel to protect it. I took a picture of it, and the 11"x14" photograph hangs on my living room wall, just in case I still have any friends who haven't heard the story yet. In the past, this award was reserved for doctors and researchers, so we were doubly honored.

My mother took care of and supported brothers and nieces and nephews through their ordeals with Huntington's Disease. She also touched countless HD families for many years as the president of the Iowa Chapter of the Committee to Combat Huntington's Disease, which later became the Huntington's Disease Society of America. In my family, besides my mother, two of my uncles had the gene and died with Huntington's Disease, and I have five cousins who now have it. I am thankful that although she was only fifty-eight when she died, she didn't have to suffer with HD. But in the back of my mind, I will wonder, "Would we have a cure now, if she were alive?"

Two wonderful genetic counselors from Iowa City continually send people going through the test to me for support and comfort. They thank me for all my help and praise me, although I don't know why. I am not smart enough to be a doctor or a researcher. I can't find the cure. But I believe since I don't have the gene, I have to make life as bearable as I can for those who do. That really seems so inadequate for all that needs to be done.

Many times all I do is listen, because that is all I can do. I have no answers, but I pray for the answers to come soon.

He Made All the Difference

BY TOM GILLIHAN

I think my sister-in-law summed it up best when she said, "It's so hard to find a doctor who is also a human being." But that is what our doctor was for us right until Helen's death. Knowing there was no cure, Dr. Byron Hanson's primary goal was to make her as comfortable as possible, and to make things as easy for our family as he could. He is a true friend as well as a great doctor.

When we first went to his office, we both liked him immediately. He seemed a little young, but was very congenial. Right off the bat, I noticed he didn't mind taking the time to really listen, and tried to answer all our questions. When Helen first started having physical difficulties a few years ago, he was very concerned and did everything he could to find out what the problem was. After we found out it was Huntington's Disease, he told us he had never had a patient with HD, but would help all he could. And that is exactly what he did.

Whenever I found new information, or specific medications that might be helpful, I brought them to Dr. Hanson. He was glad to receive what I gave him, and very interested in learning more. Unlike most doctors these days, he always had time for us. As Helen started to decline at a more rapid pace, she had many symptoms, both physical and mental. No matter what the problem, the doctor was always ready to listen. He would try to help by sending her to specialists. Or trying different medications. Or whatever it took to make life a little easier for Helen and me.

Helen liked the monthly visits to see him because he always made her feel so special. Even when it was impossible to understand her, he would always hold her hand and talk directly to her, and not just to me about her. I know it had to be very frustrating for him as we tried different medications to find a combination that would work. And I'm sure he must have gotten tired of me calling him at home and at the office; but he never showed it and kept encouraging me to call anytime we needed him.

There are doctors and scientists around the world working on finding the cure for HD. In their own way, I guess they are heroes in the fight. But to me, Dr. Hanson is just as much a hero. Maybe even more.

Huntington's Disease is just the most awful disease I can imagine. It robs humans of all their abilities. It turns them into different people and makes the world a scary place. If you let it, HD will also rob them of more. My goal throughout this was for Helen to be treated with dignity and respect. Thanks to this man, who cared enough for Helen to attend her funeral, my goal was met. Helen was treated with dignity and respect by this wonderful man who cared enough to dispense much more than drugs. He dispensed kindness, and I will forever be grateful to Dr. Hanson, my hero.

∼

Thank You, Jill

BY MARSHA INSTONE

My husband and I met Jill at an annual picnic that has been held for the last six years. This event is for the members of the North and South Carolina Huntington's Disease community. The Knucholls-Lowe Reunion is dedicated to two individuals who died with this devastating disease.

Jill Alam is the Director of HD Services for South Carolina and North Carolina, and in my eyes, she is a hero.

HD has touched her personally through the death of her affected husband and many people she has loved. It was our first in-person meeting with Jill and her family, though we met in cyberspace where I bonded with her instantly. We had chatted many times on-line and also on the phone, but this would be our first real meeting. I was so excited that I was finally going to meet my cyber buddy Jill and the people in her life that I had come to know through her conversations.

I had one of the most inspirational weekends of my life. Not only is Jill a human dynamo, but she is as beautiful on the outside as she is on the inside. Her devotion to HD, and the people affected by it, showed on every happy smiling face at that picnic. Despite the personal adversities suffered by all who attended that day, I have never met such an upbeat group of people. I know that a lot of that is due to the wonderful job that Jill has done, and the compassion and love that she gives to each one of them.

On the drive back to Ohio, I had a lot of time to think about what I had learned and witnessed that weekend. I kept catching myself with a huge smile on my face and a very warm heart thinking about all the wonderful new friends I'd made. Jill's positive attitude and caring spirit encourages me, and fills me with the hope that I will make it through whatever the next hurdle is in this battle. Whenever I am down and feel like HD is getting the best of me, all I have to do is think back to that weekend at Jill's, and my mood changes immediately. Thank you, Jill, for being you, and for continuing to fight the good fight.

Another Kind of Hero

BY GINNY SILVER-KOPOLO

Pam is my beautiful daughter. Huntington's Disease may have made her all but unrecognizable. But to me, Pam is still my beautiful daughter.

She resides in a nursing home where there are others who have HD. Pam has lost a great deal of weight, and I was called by the facility and told that, at this point, she needs a feeding tube. After the initial shock of the inevitable, I said that I had to confer with my sons, Glenn and Ricky, to see if we wanted her to have the tube. Pam can no longer walk, talk or do much of anything now. But, contrary to what many think, she is alert and aware. When we discuss things of interest around her, she attempts to chime in, or you can see her interest in the intensity of her eyes.

After a difficult discussion, her brothers and I decided that Pam had suffered long enough and it was time for her to have peace, for the suffering to end. I told the administrators that I did not want the feeding tube. I knew that I was in for a fight as the home is a privately run Catholic facility.

I began to position myself for this fight by having my husband contact my attorneys. My cousin did a lot of calling on the telephone to find out about hospice here, and it seems there are only four hospice programs in the tri-state area. I spoke to one and she was very helpful and informative, although she informed me that they only took patients with two weeks left to live. Another cousin is an influential man and on the board of directors of Brookdale Hospital in New York City. Although they do not have a hospice, he was going to call in some favors for Pam, to see what could be done.

That weekend I spent crying hysterically as I moved along doing what had to be done. As I was at the end of my emotional rope, my cousin Reggi was coordinating the family efforts, and my dear friends on-line were keeping my head together by sending messages of encouragement.

By Monday, I was an emotional wreck. Over the years, I had been asked if Pam ever had stated what she would want in a situation like this. Hospice asked the same question. Years ago, when we had never even heard of HD, Pam, as the rest of us, had said that she never wanted extraordinary measures like a feeding tube if anything ever happened to her. A little part in the corner of my mind said that was then, this is now. When someone is staring the Grim Reaper in the face, frequently they have a change of mind. I decided that I must do the unthinkable. I must ask my beautiful daughter if she wanted to die.

Glenn and I visited Pam on Monday evening. Fortunately, Liz, one of the aides who has known Pam since she entered the facility, was with her. We closed the door and told Pam that she had lost too much weight and needed the feeding tube. Looking at my beautiful daughter, I asked, "Do you want it?" She said no.

I then explained to her that if she did not get it, she would go to Grandma and God and would die. You could see her eyes intense with thought. "Do you want the tube if it is the only way you can live?" She said yes.

We asked her three different ways so that we were sure she understood us, and we understood her. It was very difficult to understand, but among the three of us, we were absolutely certain of her desires. We will respect them, because Pam is not ready to die.

Pam has had her feeding tube inserted and is doing well. The procedure is not that big a deal, but the loss of independence of eating, and the emotional loss, is devastating. The alternative was, of course, more devastating. The alternative was death.

I don't think we ever really know what our loved ones in this position want, even if he or she told you when they were in good condition. If they are at all aware, and many of them are very, very aware, as is Pam, they deserve to make the decision between life and death for themselves.

Although I hate the feeding tube, Pam wants to live. I see so little quality of life for her, but who am I to say what quality consists of? Maybe when she hears my footsteps in the hall, or some other small pleasure that the healthy take for granted, that is quality enough to keep on living.

∽

A Mother to Four
BY PAT PILLIS

My inability to have a child had left me feeling somehow empty. No matter what I did have in life, there was always the lingering sadness that I would not be a mother. Besides that loss, my first husband and I were both alcoholics, though neither one of us acknowledged our sickness. Our drinking made our lives tumultuous and things were less than pretty in our marriage. In the spring of 1981, feeling very empty, I went on what I call my spiritual quest. I now know I was looking for God; I guess I'd been doing that for years, but just hadn't realized it. I was truly looking for love in all the wrong places. I traveled extensively by myself and when I returned home to Lake Placid, NY, I began visiting Christian churches. In September of 1981, I asked Jesus Christ into my heart as my Savior. I knew I was saved, but didn't really want to change my lifestyle. Other than church attendance, I continued my less than Christian ways.

In the midst of getting on with my life, my husband and I got a phone call that there were three boys whose parents were both terminally ill. The agency was desperately seeking a new home for the children. At first, it sounded overwhelming, but we decided to go to Washington County, NY, where the boys were in foster care, and learn more about the children. That was the first time we ever heard of Huntington's Disease. Their mother was unable to care for them because she was in the late stages of HD, and their father was dying from emphysema. We knew that the boys were at-risk, but we were also assured that most people did not get the disease until they were well into adulthood. I prayed as I'd never prayed before, and the Lord seemed to say, "It's not their fault." I had asked my church family, beginning in January 1984, to pray for a baby for us. One Sunday in March of 1984, I brought all three boys to church and said, "Please stop praying."

Our new sons were ten, six and two and had been named Fred, Kevin, and Shane respectively. They had a fourth brother, Michael, who had been adopted out of the family before I met them. On the day they came home, my drinking progressed to being a daily occurrence. I had no idea how to take care of them, so I stuck my head in the ground with my bottle. They came with more baggage than I had realized. Even now I am still learning about how long we carry our baggage with us and how devastating it can be. I let them know that we each had a job. Their job was school and day care, and that was that.

On May 4, 1986, thanks to comments made by my oldest son, and being sick and tired of being sick and tired, I found my way into sobriety. By the grace of God, I am still sober today and that is a real trick, considering we are now looking at HD head on. My husband and drinking buddy was not thrilled about my sobriety, so a little over a year later, we separated and I kept the boys. We moved to Saranac Lake because Shane was having serious behavior problems and the school district was better able to care for special needs students. I believe that was the beginning of our family struggles with Huntington's Disease.

While I fought to stay sober, and the boys worked on having normal lives, we put HD on the back burner. We visited the boys' parents on occasion, eventually attending their funerals. Fred, who had been taught a physically violent way of dealing with life by his birth dad, ended up moving in with my ex-husband because of his violence and large size. At fourteen, he was an angry six-foot-two-inch adolescent, compared to my five-foot-two-inch frame.

In 1989, social services contacted me because they had a baby that turned out to be my little Shannon. I had always dreamed of having a daughter, but had given up that hope when I became a single mother. I believe that God worked a miracle by bringing her into our lives. She was fourteen months old at the time, and here I was, a single mom, about to take on more. Of course, people thought I was crazy, and maybe I was. But I also know I was blessed. Now I had four children and loved them all dearly, so life continued with HD still on the back burner.

In June 1990, I married my second husband, Paul Pillis. When I was divorced, there were two things of which I was certain. I knew I would never have my little girl, and there was no man on this earth that was going to come along and marry me with all these not-so-easy kids. What I didn't realize, and still forget at times, is that I serve the God of the impossible. Kevin and Shane gave me away at our wedding, and so began another phase of life.

All went beautifully well until the summer of 1991,

when Kevin decided, at age fourteen, to move in with his dad in Lake Placid. My heart was shattered, and it was a rocky time in our family life. He has since returned and lives part time with us and part time with his dad while he attends college. We have a great relationship now, but then it was very difficult.

During these years, Shane was diagnosed with Attention Deficit Hyperactive Disorder, put on Ritalin, and was always in special education classes. He was an excellent academic student, but behavior was always a problem with him. He was never mean, simply out of control and inappropriate. Three or four years ago, as he entered early adolescence, Shane's behavior started getting worse. We chalked some of it up to being a teenager. He was not maturing as other kids, and seemed to be losing the few friends he had. There were times when he was sexually inappropriate for his age as well. With each year he got worse, and finally I asked the doctors about the possibility of HD, but was told he was too young.

Then the stealing began. He broke into friends' homes when they vacationed and started swearing uncontrollably when he was angry, which was often. My heart broke for him, and I did not react well. Paul and I started arguing about Shane's behavior. He insisted Shane had gone bad and needed to be turned over to the police, while I was convinced that he still had a sweet nature and was just sick.

Through it all, we visited neurologists, who said he just had a tic, and psychologists, who said he was a tough case and unreachable. School districts tried to be supportive but were baffled by him, and pastors encouraged more prayer. When none of those strategies worked, we had him admitted to Four Winds Psychiatric Hospital in Saratoga Springs on March 10, 1997. A few days after he arrived, they gave him Depacote, and he went totally insane. They tried a number of other medications over the next few days but they all had the same effect. For eight days, he was placed in isolation and was in a constant rage. It was terrifying. He was finally taken off all medication, and some sort of therapy began for him. We were running the roads between home and the hospital about two times each week. The expense of the two-hour drive as well as loss of work time for my husband began to take a toll financially. But we knew Shane had to be the priority at this stage. In the midst of this, poor Shannon was in tears in my room with an innate knowledge that things at home would never be the same again.

In April, the psychiatrist at Four Winds, in conjunction with a neurologist from Glens Falls, finally diagnosed Shane with HD. Rivers of tears have been shed since that time. Although in my heart I had suspected HD for years, to hear the actual words was still a shock. Shane came home on April 18, knowing that he has this awful monster of a disease. Though he knows he is dying from it, he is in denial and believes he will live to be sixty, have children, and live a full life as a wealthy inventor. His sweet innocence helps him cope. As a family, we continue to draw closer to one another and to God, and we have had many healing prayer times together and with friends. I believe that Shane has been healed in his spirit and in his anger, though the HD rages on in its devastating way.

Kevin and Fred live under the shadow of their at-risk status. Kevin has begun the process of deciding whether to be tested, but Fred chooses not to be tested at this time. Their fourth brother, Michael, who was abandoned by his adoptive family when he started with the outrageous behavior in high school, is now twenty-two and has Huntington's Disease. We are drawing him into our family circle as much as he'll let us.

We all live with this disease the same way Paul and I live with alcoholism; one day at a time. We try not to project too much into the future, and Shane gets us laughing often when situations arise that could make us cry. We have started visiting long-term care facilities to help us choose an appropriate home for him, if it does become necessary to have him taken care of outside the home at some future date. We try not to plan when or why, but to trust God to let us know.

Shane had the genetic test recently, and with a CAG* repeat of sixty-four, it served to confirm the diagnosis and somewhat explain his early onset. We pray daily for a cure, and often donate to researchers so they can continue the fight. It may not come soon enough for our Shane, but it might for others out there who are pre-symptomatic like Kevin and Fred. People often ask me if I knew they were at-risk when I adopted them. Not only did I know, but I would do it again. It kept them together as brothers and I love them as my own. We need support of friends and family as never before, and I just pray that people don't reject Shane as his good looks deteriorate.

I believe that I was hand-picked to be a mother to my children while learning valuable lessons at the same time. I have had many struggles before and after the diagnosis of Huntington's Disease. However, living a life with HD has helped me to grow more trusting of God, more compassionate of others in need, and has given me a larger capacity to love.

---

* CAG are the names of DNA nucleotides, Cytosine/Adenosine/Guanosine.

A Chance Encounter

BY MURRAY DANIEL THOMPSON

My connection with Huntington's Disease began as a chance encounter. As a young man at the university, I found it necessary to both study and work to meet expenses. I'd left my previous employment, and enrolled to undertake a degree in Physiotherapy, known in some places as Physical Therapy.

I answered an advertisement in the daily paper for a job involving care for people with HD. I knew nothing of the disease or its processes, and was purely looking for some part time work that would also allow me time to study. Undaunted by my ignorance of HD, I interviewed with an institution in Melbourne, Australia. Then, it was the only center of its kind in the world dedicated exclusively to the care of those with HD. At my interview, I was asked, "Do you know what HD is?" I replied in ignorance, "Yes, my grandfather has it." You see, as others have done, I had mistaken HD for Hodgekin's Disease.

The interview ended, and I was asked to find out for sure what disease my grandfather was suffering from, and get back to them. With some embarrassment I let them know of my error. I later realized they were protecting me. Imagine exposing someone who was potentially at-risk of inheriting the disease to the reality of the symptoms, if they knew nothing of the disease. However, as my grandfather did not have HD, the interview went well and I started work soon thereafter.

My first day, even my first minute, was, to say the least, a shock. I'd never been in an institution before. My initial contact was with the strong smell of urine, moaning, shrieking, screaming and of people wandering, stumbling.

My discomfort was increased because the residents were quite demanding of the staff. Many of the patients looked disfigured; twisted, thin and often unkempt. There was very little interaction with many of them. They just seemed to be sitting and lying around. I was curious, and I suppose horrified, in a low key sort of way. The chorea and grimacing were the most disconcerting, but I felt myself wanting to know more about these people and how they were suffering.

Before long, I had worked quite a number of shifts, and the individual personalities began to emerge. The horror was hidden by smiles, laughter, charity, and strong independent wills, and a respect was born in me that was greater than just a professional ethic. My work, although basically menial, gave me time to look into the emotional side of those I was caring for, and I began to forge some good relationships with many of the residents. But as time went on, I began to feel that very little could be done for these people. All manner of comfort and convenience and activity was attempted, but in all, they seemed doomed.

As their symptoms progressed, their difficulties with daily tasks increased, and their poor communication left them with more frustration. As my interaction progressed, I felt I really needed to try to do more for these people. It was the small things that they missed most. Finding that favorite pair of shoes, or going to the safe for someone so they could wear their pearls for the day if they wanted to was important. Consideration for their desires and passions was vital. To me, much of the staff was stressed, overworked; it seemed they were there because this was the only work available to them.

My studies progressed well, and I began studying neurosciences and neuroanatomy. Thus, I began to understand the pathology of HD more. I also looked more at what else could better help them and we tried exercise, music, communication boards, and even supervised horse riding. There was, and still is, a small, dedicated group of health professionals working with HD. There were always some new ideas coming forward and being expressed in the hope that they would enhance someone's life and leisure. But overall, we knew our limitations, the reality of the disease, and its progression.

Staff turnover was high, perhaps because of burn out, and it was only a few years until I was among the senior, most experienced staff. People frequently asked me about managing certain emotional issues because I knew the residents and their personalities so well. Unfortunately, I also witnessed the progression of HD in many of the people, and the passing of quite a few; I watched them battle the falls and injuries, immobility, dysphagia and choking, respiratory compromise and isolation. There seemed to be so little going on in some of the people; I wondered what they were thinking, where they went in their dreams. Yet, taking the residents for granted was a mistake. They often dazzled you with their memory, insight and recognition. Once I took a patient to the Australian Tennis Open. Bruce, who had not spoken clearly in months, shouted at the top of his voice so all could hear in the stadium, "Come on, Monica!" I was surprised as he hadn't spoken clearly for some months. I can't recall if Monica Seles won that match. If she did, maybe she has Bruce to thank.

The thing that stood out most about HD and the people it affects is that human personality burns through, even to the end of the disability; enjoyment of life and pleasure are fundamental rights, yet sometimes people who are around them much think that their disease limits their ability to enjoy themselves. Another thing that stood out was that HD crossed all the boundaries of education and experience. I knew of people from every economic and educational class. HD marched through all their lives with the same disastrous effects. For some, death seems to be a satisfying curtain to the suffering, discomfort and indignities of the disease.

One lady I knew well fought HD for over ten years, with spite and screaming and lashing out at staff. At thirty-five kilograms, Marie was a frail, tiny woman, a spinster with only a few family friends. She had one brother who had managed to escape HD. Marie had favorite shoes and would call out "Footrest, Footrest" when being dressed. This was the name of the brand of her shoes. If you listened you could make out what she wanted, but many workers just grabbed whatever was handy. To find the favorites and pop on those shoes made her very satisfied and content. It was the least we could do, and simple, but it gave Marie some control over her life. Allowing people a measure of control where possible is an important factor we miss sometimes. I gave Marie all the time I could. She rarely thanked me; she just didn't hit me. All of her independence had been lost over the years, and I felt she was embarrassed by herself and her life and predicament. Marie's life was a burden to herself, but there were times when the chorea would settle a little and she did seem at peace. I rather feel at these times after fighting, screaming and being anxious for hours she was more exhausted than anything else.

I saw Marie almost every day for almost six years. During that time, I did my best to help her cope with HD. I did feel that Marie trusted me and when I talked, she'd often laugh about certain things, seeing the irony in many of my offerings. She could really only respond with "Yes" and "No," but strong dislikes were always met with arm actions, like pushing food away violently. I suspect this was the result of being fed food that was often way too hot.

There were several times when Marie's health deteriorated so that we thought she would die. But, to our surprise, she would rally and battle on again. In the end, during my last year at the center, I arrived one afternoon and found Marie in a sitting room with fifteen others. No one was communicating; just sitting in front of the TV staring into space. Marie looked gaunt, with eyes sunken – and in respiratory distress. The irregularity of her breathing and lack of response were strong signs to me that Marie was dying very quickly. I couldn't let her go like this, in a public room, in front of all those blank eyes.

Grabbing the nurse in charge, he and I took Marie into her room with its quietude. She died in my arms. At sixty-two years of age, and a mere fraction of what she should have weighed, she was seemingly just burnt out with the disease. Her body was limp and without chorea, the first time since I had known her. What a sad thing, I thought, that Marie might have died alone, without anyone to care at her end. I was glad to be able to offer her my arms in that final moment. I had not seen anyone die before and I was sad. But I was full of respect for how Marie had battled and struggled with HD for so long without rest, until she let it go. It also burned an impression, that no one deserves to die alone.

HD has changed my life, and although I have a lot less to do with the disease nowadays, I still find myself talking about it with other health professionals. I am actively involved with the Australian Huntington's Disease Association in training their new staff in the role of Physiotherapy with HD. Through all things, no matter how terrible, we must take hold of the positive. Seeing the perseverance of people with Huntington's Disease, and the strength of family and caregivers, we see that the human spirit overcomes all things in time.

To Pitta

BY LEON JOFFE

You surprise me every day –
Your fighting spirit
Your vision and its ability to draw me forward with you
Your loveliness even as you plunge through the hard core of
our future

You achieve what others dare not even dream about
You know no barriers to the universe
You are my dreamer, my leader
With you I am greater than myself
With you I can carry my perpetual fear that sits inside me
like a rock
Turned by you to water
To drain away through the tunnel of your laughter and
courage

This day we face together another challenge
I here too distant to do more than love you

I will myself to weakness
That my strength may add to yours
I will myself to passivity
That your actions may shame and humble all like me

Know then how much I admire you
And much more than that,
Love you

~ 11

Chuck's Story

BY CHUCK YOUNG

ALL my life I have been the strong one. I'm from Texas, and you know how Texan men are – larger than life, good providers and we never cry.

For all that, though, this Texan's heart melted when I saw Linda at the Valentine's banquet, when we were both in the eighth grade. That was our first date. Although there were high school flirtations with others, neither of us ever dated anyone else. After one year of college, Linda became Mrs. Young and we began our life together.

We were both disappointed when tests finally showed I was unable to have children, but of course, now we know that was a blessing. Our disappointment turned to joy when in 1968, we received the most special present of that or any Christmas since. Four-day-old Michelle entered our home and our hearts through the miracle of adoption. Life just couldn't get any better.

Our little family settled into our routine, going through similar trials and joys of any middle class American family.

I was in the petroleum equipment business for twenty-five years, but the oil crunch in the mid-1980s ended that career. It also wiped out all of our financial assets. But we were young, and so in 1986, I began selling Life Insurance, Retirement Planning, Disability Insurance, and Long Term Care. Our financial situation again prospered, and then my Michelle announced she was going to make me the proudest grandpa in Texas. Little Cayley, that stands for my initials, CAY, and Linda's initials LEY, was to be the beginning of what we just knew would be the best stage of our lives. Boy, were we wrong.

In May of 1990, Linda decided to take a series of golf lessons. One of her main problems was that she could not keep her feet still while she hit the ball. While she was addressing and hitting the ball, her feet kept shifting. Linda has never in her life dealt well with pressure and I teased her a little about keeping her feet still. I realized that just the pressure of taking the lessons made her nervous.

Over the next year or so, every time she sat down, she would kick her feet until her shoes would come off. I also noticed that she was wearing out her shoes in record time. The upper part of her shoes were badly scuffed and torn. As time continued, the foot twitching became leg kicking. She explained to me that the reason she was wearing out her shoes so quickly was that she kicked them on her secretarial chair at work.

During this time, she also became very emotional, impulsive, and anxious about everything. Coupled with her anxiety was the stress of rebuilding our financial security, the normal stress of living in today's society, the marriage of our daughter, and just the experience of moving into our fifties.

Linda expressed that she felt as if she had a motor running inside her that she couldn't control. I suggested to her that since she was experiencing the change of life, she should express this feeling to her gynecologist. She did, but she was basically ignored. I then suggested she talk with our family doctor about this, and again, there was not much response.

Being the determined person I am, early in 1992, I said we were going to find out what was going on regardless of what it took. We were referred to a neurologist here in Amarillo, but after our first visit, we both came out angry. He didn't listen to what we told him, but instead, seemed to have his own agenda. He said he wasn't sure what the problem was, but named a string of diseases that could be the culprit. Without even having a diagnosis, he gave us a prescription of Haldol and told us to come back in six months. I read up on Haldol and it scared me to death, but I decided he knew a lot more than I did. So, despite my misgivings, we followed his instructions. The Haldol stripped Linda of who she was and gave her a masked face, no emotions; she became a very drugged-out gal. All the while, Linda continued to work and drive.

After six months, I decided we were not going back to him and, with some direction from my company doctor in New York, went to another neurologist. He said the exact same thing as the first doctor, but he did listen, and suggested staying on the Haldol. After six months, and some progression in symptoms, my company doctor said we needed to get her to a teaching hospital or a large neurological clinic. We made an appointment with a highly qualified doctor in Dallas, Texas, which is three hundred sixty-two miles from Amarillo.

This doctor put Linda through the tests and said she wasn't sure about the problem, but took her off her medications and gradually started her on Kolonopin. Every time we went to Dallas, the neurologist would call other neurologists in from the clinic to observe, but the elusive mystery still remained. Finally, she referred us to Dr. Jankovic of Baylor Medical School in Houston.

I knew Dr. Jankovic's name because I had asked one of the Amarillo doctors who the best neurologist in Texas was. The good news was that without hesitation he answered, "Dr. Jankovic in Houston." The bad news was that Dr. Jankovic no longer sees patients but travels world wide giving seminars and writes the books that neurologists study. When I mentioned this to the doctor in Dallas, she said that she had done a fellowship under Dr. Jankovic and he would see Linda. In less than a month, Linda and I were sitting in Dr. Jankovic's office.

After a brief neurological exam, he said, "I think the problem is Huntington's Disease, but we can find out with a blood test." After all this time, I could not believe something so simple as a blood test was available. The blood was taken that day in October of 1995. He also filmed Linda walking and they performed an MRI.

On December 15, 1995, at 12:00 noon, six months before Cayley was born, I entered the house; Linda was standing in the middle of the living room with her arms outstretched, waiting for a hug. The first thing she said was, "Dr. Jankovic called me this morning and my Huntington's test was positive." We hugged and cried for a while, and I said, "Well, at least now we know."

We really didn't have a hint about what was ahead for us, because we had never heard of Huntington's. A couple of the other neurologists had said that what she had could be Wilson's, Huntington's, Tourette's, or Restless Leg. We thought HD was just one more disease to rule out. We had never seen anyone with this awful disease either, and we knew nothing about it. Oh, to be that naive again.

Although I had been trying to get Linda to quit work

for about two years, she kept saying that if they could find the problem and correct it, she wanted to continue working. The probable diagnosis spelled the end of her career, and her last day of work was October 22, 1995. For several months before she quit, we would come home and lie on the bed for an hour or more before she felt like eating dinner. This was a difficult time for her, she didn't feel like doing anything around the house. That bothered her so much because she didn't want me to do it all either. Many discussions and tears were had during this time as I was doing more and more of the cleaning, washing, shopping, and cooking when she didn't feel like it. Something in her rebelled, and she didn't want me to do it all. I kept explaining to her that since she didn't feel like doing it, she needed to just rest and allow me to handle those things. Until this time, we had always been a fifty/fifty team on housework.

Linda's father died at forty of a massive heart attack. His two sisters, Linda's aunts, had died in their twenties and thirties of cancer, and her grandfather died as a young man in a farm accident. The Thompson family was not close knit and there weren't many family members. As we quizzed Linda's mother about the Thompsons, she kept stating that there wasn't anyone else like Linda in the family. Much later, she did admit that there was one other family member that did sling her head from one side to another. Linda's father stuttered in his youth, had slow mannerisms and you could see the wheels turning long before anything was spoken. There was also a cousin who was the same.

Dr. Jankovic in Houston prescribed Tetrabenazine, which is an investigational drug. Although chorea is a primary symptom, Tetrabenazine has worked pretty well. In the summer of 1996, Linda's appetite went wild. She

233

would eat huge servings of a meal and 30 minutes later complain of being hungry. She went from one hundred thirty pounds to one hundred ninety pounds. During this period, it became impossible for her to sleep, and the less sleep she got, the more the symptoms raged on. When we brought this to the doctor's attention, he said the same part of the brain controls the eating, sleeping, and sex drive, and he prescribed Prozac to slow these symptoms. She has been on Prozac since that time and I'm convinced this is part of the reason Linda is doing as well as she is.

During the last year or so, symptoms have progressed rather steadily. Now she is unable to do anything other than eat and sleep and watch TV. Her chorea is erratic, sometimes calm and other times violent. Her ability to reason or be reasonable is almost non-existent. She is as impulsive as a young child and wants everything now. She has no patience. For example, the minute I begin preparing a meal, she wants it right now. Her balance and walking ability varies, but most of the time, she ricochets from one wall to another. She simply leans forward and just falls until she runs into something. Sometimes she eats and talks well, and other times she has a great deal of trouble with both.

Every day I experience almost every emotion known to man. I guess I will never know why God allowed such an ugly disease to consume such a beautiful lady. You see, the very first time I saw Linda was at church in the eighth grade, and I was determined that she would be my girlfriend. Little did I know that for the next forty years, she would be my best friend and companion. I guess a boy would not comprehend what that would mean, but from the age of fourteen, that is exactly the relationship we have had. We have done virtually everything as one including working, planning, laughing, crying, traveling, relaxing, playing, saving, spending, sleeping, and making love. Now, for some reason, God has allowed most of that to be taken from us. I still experience love when she calls me twenty, thirty times a day saying, "I love you." But I also realize that, at some point, hearing that will also be taken from me.

I never paid much attention to caregivers before, and I didn't understand what those words meant until the last three years. People began expressing their admiration and appreciation and concern for me, but I just brushed off their comments with a "Thank you." You see, I had always been known in our circle of friends as the strong one, the one that could fix things, the doer, the one with big shoulders. As time has progressed, I have become proud of the term caregiver, and I now appreciate what it means.

For an HD caregiver, it means giving of yourself far more than one has to give. It means having far more patience than you have ever thought possible. It means experiencing emotional mountain tops and valley lows all in one day. It means having a friend ask, "How is Linda, Chuck?" and instantly bursting out in tears, bawling like a child. Yes, the big, brave, strong Chuck may now be seen, any time and any place, with tears in his eyes from the broken heart of seeing what this ugly disease has done to the one he loves.

I think that God gave most of the ability for nursing and sympathizing to the female. Men and women are different and this is one of the differences. Most of us men are the hunters, providers, and warriors. The men I know, including myself, don't have what it takes to feel comfortable being a caregiver. But when faced with the necessity, I think I do a good job.

Linda and I have always been active. We have always enjoyed going places and doing things together. Unlike most men, I didn't go to the ball games with the guys, I went with Linda. For the first two years that Linda was immobilized, I stayed home with her all the weekends and evenings. I got to the point, though, that I had to "break out,"so to speak. I finally became aware that Linda was going to be this way for a long time and I still had the need to go to the ball games and car races. I had to get away by myself to take my mind off everything. I have, over the last year or so, found ways and places to go for a Friday or Saturday evening of escape from the reality of our lives. When I first started doing this, I felt guilty, and many times would leave at half time because I felt I should be at home. I have learned to enjoy this free time and don't feel guilty anymore. I enjoy my private time but I would still prefer having the company of my little lady.

I just placed Linda in a nursing home, which I did with a heart full of love. She will have better and more constant care than I can give her because of my working. Her eighty-one-year-old mother had been very helpful, providing much of Linda's care, and the cleaning, cooking, and laundry. Her help allowed me to keep Linda home longer than otherwise.

So many emotions are going through my soul right now; sadness, loneliness, fear, anger, and, yes, even relief. Her mother and I just couldn't deal physically or emotionally with caring for her. Her mother said, "No one would understand unless they have cared for a person with Huntington's Disease."

Linda is content, and okay with the move. As I left the first time, she said, "Dad, I'm going to like it here." Who knows why she would say something like that. Yes, it is a pleasant place, but that comment really grabbed me.

I checked her in on a Wednesday and she was having her best day in weeks. I went back Thursday, and she was the same; just as happy as she could be. There was very little chorea, no choking, no vomiting. I went back Friday, and I knew it wasn't a fluke; she was happy and comfortable. I asked the social worker (Christy) what was going on, why the massive change? She said she had talked with Linda, and this was her explanation.

"She is eating more nourishing food," the social worker explained. "At home you fixed what she wanted, rather than what was good for her."

I told her that when I fixed healthy foods, she wouldn't eat them.

"Yes," Christy said. "But she is eating everything on her tray, and sometimes seconds. The sociability aspect is also good. She is around new people, and she has people checking on her and taking care of her other than her mother and husband. You have taken the stress out of her life."

I asked her what she meant by the stress. Christy explained, "She doesn't worry whether you will be there at 12:00 or 12:05. Also, she hated the fact that you were having to take care of her, clean up the various messes she made, take care of the house, and work."

I told Christy that she often apologized, and my standard answer was, "Linda, it's not your fault." Christy said Linda understood, but she still felt awful about it. Christy also said Linda told her she could be "a better wife at the nursing home than she could be at home." That truly brought me to tears.

All this time, I thought placing Linda in a nursing home was wrong. I guess each situation is different. We are both as content as possible, and her symptoms are back like they were about a year ago. I told my pastor if anyone visited that didn't know what she was like, it would almost be embarrassing. They would wonder why she is in a nursing home.

I still pray daily for a cure for this ugly disease. Although Linda has probably progressed beyond where a cure would help, I would love to live in a world where no one would ever suffer as Linda and I and countless others have.

12

Faces of Faith

BY CARMEN LEAL-POCK

T*here is a reason for all things. Faith means we don't always have to have the answer.*

—Petey Parker

There is a story I once heard about two artists. I never forgot it because of the impact it made on me.

Around the year 1490, there were two young friends, Albrecht Durer and Franz Knigstein, both very poor, struggling artists. So poor, they had to work to support themselves while they studied.

As eager as they were both to perfect their craft, their work took so much of their time, there were few moments left for art. Finally, they agreed to a plan. If one of them could study exclusively, he would surely become successful. The one who achieved such fame would then pay for the other friend to study. After drawing lots, Albrect began his education, while Franz supported them both.

Albrect went off to the cities of Europe to learn. As predicted, he did attain that elusive success, and, as promised, went back to keep his vow to Franz. It was when Albrecht returned home to Franz that he saw the enormous cost his friend had paid.

While Albrect had spent his time learning and drawing, Franz had done manual labor to provide for him. His fingers had become stiff and gnarled; his artists' hands were ruined for life. But although his dreams would never be realized, he was not bitter. Instead, he rejoiced at all his friend had achieved.

One day, Albrecht came to his friend and found him kneeling, with his twisted hands positioned in prayer. Franz was praying for his friend, though he himself could no longer be an artist. Albrecht Durer sketched the folded hands of his faithful friend and later completed his greatest masterpiece, "The Praying Hands."

As I reflect on the story surrounding the painting, I realize this picture is not just a finely crafted piece of artwork, it is a story of love, encouragement, and, yes, faith.

Wanting to engage him in the companionable conversations we used to share, I have often asked my husband what he thinks about each day.

"Oh, stuff," he replies.

"What kind of stuff?"

He smiles and says, "I pray." "

"What do you pray about?" He never answers that he prays for himself. Instead he prays for my success in writing, or for my children to do well in school and in their future endeavors. He asks God to make my life a little easier and to provide all we need. He prays for others in his life, even for those who have seemingly forgotten him.

I once asked Dave if he ever got mad at God.

His response was, "Why should I be mad at God?" He said that God gave him an incredibly wonderful life. He prays instead that God's will is done, and that he has the faith to accept that will. I am humbled by his expression of love for me; it reminds me of the two young artists.

For some people, faith is the belief that God is real and that He will ultimately do what is right. For others, faith is another word for positive thinking. I think that, regardless of a person's definition of faith, when real faith happens, a mind set is developed that looks for the best in everything. Such faith often results from a crisis that has happened.

Dave and I saw a movie recently where everything kept going wrong for two hapless fishermen. All they wanted in life was to fish, and they won a fishing trip that was going to be incredible. As happens in movies, and often in life, the trip was a disaster with calamity following crisis. One character would get depressed and angry and talk about how awful the trip was. The other fisherman would say, "But it could be worse!" He would extol the obvious good events and downplay the catastrophes. By the time he was done, his friend would agree that maybe things weren't so bad after all. Over and over, the two men plunged from one low moment to the next, somehow managing to rise to the occasion and continue their journey.

That's faith. These two men had faith that they were going to have the best fishing trip ever. Nothing was going to get in the way, and no matter what cards they were dealt, they would play them to the best of their admittedly limited abilities. By the end of the movie, they had experienced the best time imaginable.

I sat in amazement at the way they were able to turn what to me was a horrible trip, into a shining moment in their lives. I cheered at their unflagging joy and faith. I wanted to take on their attitude and surround myself with people just like them.

Anyone who is living with Huntington's, in any way, has been dealt one of the worst imaginable blows. They have every reason to lose faith and feel as if they have been cheated. But when we have faith, our quality of life is improved. The belief that somehow everything will work out, that we are not doing this alone, can help get us through each day in a much more optimistic, peaceful frame of mind.

Abraham Lincoln said, "I have been driven many times to go to my knees by the overwhelming conviction that I had nowhere else to go." Mr. Lincoln is not the only one who has had that conviction. However satisfying and normal it is to have control over ourselves, our lives and our circumstances, it is comforting to hand back that control to One who orders all. Nothing could be more out of control than HD. It is good to go to our knees when things are going well and when they are not. When all hope of control is gone, we need to call on our faith.

With strengthening faith, comes peace. Peace from God does not mean that we will not give way to human emotions. Just because we may cry or feel bad does not mean that we no longer trust and have faith in God. It just means that we are acting the way God has created us to act... emotions and all.

Julie, a member of a support group, summed it up this way when she responded to a member who was sharing her problems in communicating with her recently diagnosed husband.

"Advice, I don't have... except it will improve with time. When my husband was first diagnosed, he reminded me every day that he was dying. He talked about suicide a lot of the time, how he was going to do it, where and when. If I got upset about his suicide talk, I would get about the same response as you have gotten. Something like, 'I am the one who is dying, and you only want to think of yourself.' Or, ' I'm not even really sick yet and you don't have any patience. What is it going to be like when I am?'

"We are now three years past diagnosis, and my husband no longer talks of suicide. He no longer reminds me that he is dying. He has become more supportive of me in many ways. I don't think I did anything to bring this about. I think I am the same person. My friends, however, tell me I have changed. They say that since I have been working on a better relationship with God, I am different, and that is what has affected him. Whatever, I am just thankful he is better."

∽

Trusting God
BY CARMEN LEAL-POCK

At church, the pastor asked us to pray for forgiveness that we might be ready to receive Communion. Normally, as I pray under these circumstances, I am able to recite a laundry list of sins.

On this occasion, I simply tried to still my emotions and spirit. I asked the Lord to please show me how I had saddened Him the most. He knows all my sins, He doesn't need a recital of these sins to forgive them.

As the music played gently in the background, I heard Him whisper lovingly, "You simply don't trust me, my child. Don't you know nothing is too big for me?" The silent tears began to course down my face as I realized how true this was. Yes, I have problems that seem immense to the average person. The ten thousand dollars in medical bills, no health insurance, little income, a dying husband and raising two teenagers virtually alone are gigantic problems. However, my God is not an average person. He has promised He will always provide for me.

He will always take what is evil or sad or disastrous in my life and turn it into good for His glory, because He knows I love him.

The myriad of sins I could have uttered died on my lips as I confessed the sin of not trusting God. I had somehow elevated myself to the one who has all the answers. I realized that God never asked me to solve every problem. He never asked me to be a superwoman. All God has ever asked, and will ever ask, is that I trust Him. I need to trust God in every area of my life, even when it seems He is not working things out. Because God is perfect, He is incapable of letting me down.

∽

Dear God

BY SHIRLEY PROCELL

Dear God, please help me
I feel so alone
I'm frightened and worried
Of what is unknown
But, you, precious Lord
Can calm all my fears
Your merciful grace
Will dry up my tears
I come as your child
In search of your love
And thanking you, God
For the gifts from above.

With Childlike Faith

BY LORETTA DELAUTER

When I was a little girl, I knew my parents loved me. No one had to explain it to me; I just knew. Even when my mom got sick, I still knew she loved me. I was trusting of my parents and never questioned their love. I have always believed in a God who cares for me since my childhood. Even when I didn't understand, I knew instinctively that He loved me and only wanted what was best for me. I still have that faith, and because we had no religious instruction at home, I know my faith is a true gift from Him.

Along with that faith, I have been blessed throughout my life with joy and optimism; turning a bad situation into a good one has become part of my style of living. When I was five years old, my mom entered a nursing home because she had Huntington's Disease. She went to heaven ten years later. Losing my mom when I was fifteen taught me how precious life is; I try to thank God every day for all my blessings, and for the simple things of life.

My childhood was full of hurts and traumas. I often felt God was the only one I could really trust. God continued to assure me of His love by putting a wonderful lady in my life; a mother figure who was like an angel sent from heaven.

While working on my nursing degree, I came across patients with Huntington's Disease. Of course, I was full of questions. I went to my father about my mother's death, and this is when I found out what HD was, and that my siblings and I had a chance of getting the disease.

A year after graduation, I got engaged to a terrific man who had attended a Lutheran church all his life. Before we married, my dad told him all about HD, and what could happen. However, my husband also has faith. He is an optimist. We married as planned, and joined a Lutheran church together. Within three years, we had out first child and moved to Frederick County.

In 1994, a son joined our family. He has had problems with asthma since he was two months old, but I have found no matter the trials, God is always right there beside us. When I allow God to work, He will do wonders, and He has. The pastor and our church have been a real blessing to us as well.

I was diagnosed with HD in March of 1995. I've always had a gut feeling that I had it, so when I went through the genetic testing process, I felt as if I already knew the answer. Again, I trusted God to take care of my husband, my kids, and me. Since that time, I have felt like I want to live each second, minute, hour, and day the way God would want me to.

As of today, there is no cure for HD. I know there are those who question how I can rejoice in my trials, and how I can have faith that God really does love me. I guess for me, I focus on the most important things... and HD doesn't happen to be the most important thing in my life. My relationship with Jesus, and helping my children to have faith in Him as well, is all-important to me. I want them to be able to turn to God for all their needs. To that end I have started a prayer journal so I can share my faith, and how God has been there for me over and over. If the time comes when I am not able to tell or show my children about my faith, my journal will speak volumes. I want my children to be able to see people through Jesus' eyes; even those who act different or stumble and fall and look drunk.

HD has been a blessing in that it has made my faith grow, and in turn, has made me into a stronger person. I don't hide facts about HD as some people do. Instead, everyone in my church is well aware of my future and what to expect. I have gotten into a Bible Study, Sunday School and more fellowship with friends who pray for me on a regular basis. I get more comfort from the power of prayer, and my faith, than anything else.

As for the future, there is always the hope of intervention or a cure. However, I don't really worry or fear the unknown. I trust God because He knows what is best. I need to continually draw on that childlike faith. It is this faith, coupled with prayer, that gives me the strength and hope to carry on.

Heart For Any Fate (Psalm)

BY Bruce P., Miami, Fl

Which God picks so aimlessly from our family tree,
Who is next, you or me?
Dare we ask how or why?
How to live, when to die?

Do not look down on us, Lord, mercilessly,
lost in this genetic maelstrom.
Toss me not into the night forlorn.
To Thy allegiance I have sworn.

Whose fate awaits me now, Lord, my mother's
muscular mess, who preferred death and peace to her plight;
Please, Oh Lord, choose not for me her dark night.

Come now and forever, Oh Lord. Find a miraculous end to this pall.
Please stay this tragic end for all.
Cast from our house this quivering, shaking gene
that takes our Woodies (Guthrie), that makes us
shudder in fear from birth, that robs us of half of our lives,
and makes us wish that we had never been born.

Do you need me for this experiment, Oh Lord?

We need this miracle now, Oh Lord. Please not another minute wait,
That I may not walk my mother's gait.
Send it, Lord, in today's mail,
that we no longer hear a graveside wail.

If this Eternal Covenant shall be,
then let us walk straight and free.
Let us not come home to a vacant chair,
or another black patch to wear, our sorrow too great to bear.
Console us now,
Visit us now,
Save us now.

Do not let our naked heart beat alone for too long.
We beg Thee, Oh Lord, cast off our crutches, set us right.
Let us not have another long, endless night.
Let us see
That is why we come to Thee.

A Prayer

BY JEAN E. MILLER

Dear God in heaven, up above
I've come to talk to you about Huntington's
and what it does to those we love.

It takes these people, once so innocent,
steals their speech and abilities to function
leaving them frustrated, feeling hopelessly spent.

Then it hurts those who have them in their care
stretching their pockets, hearts and good will
Sometimes it is more than their faith can bear.

And then there are those who turn away
breaking your teachings to help one another
causing them to wander and stray.

There are some who say that you are only testing
That you will never give more than we can handle
Are you watching, God, and giving us your blessing?

The strength comes through our belief in your love
that helps us through the darkness of night
When our very souls cry out for help from you, above.

Oh, please dear God, help those once so pure
to rediscover our faith unresolved
And if it wouldn't be too much, send us a cure.

Dr. Huntington, I Presume?

BY GREG

On June 4, 1997, my wife and I approached the genetics clinic with a mixed sense of nervousness and optimism. Despite our anxiety, we were both excited to receive the long awaited results of the genetic test. We took our seats after being ushered into the office, and the doctor turned to us.

"How are you feeling?" she asked.

"Nervous," we responded almost in unison.

"Do you want to receive the results?" she asked me.

"Yes," I croaked response.

She slowly lifted a piece of paper, glanced down and then back into my eyes, "I'm sorry, but you have the gene and will one day develop Huntington's Disease."

I was thunderstruck; it felt utterly surreal. I glanced at my weeping wife and the entire scenario being played out was like a bad dream. How could this possibly be? At thirty-three, I had everything, a beautiful wife, a wonderful son, a company that was my own. Things had always seemed to go well for me in the overall scheme. I had the looks and the brains to get me through anything. This was too much, it just couldn't be.

As we left the hospital, my wife continued crying... then something strange happened. She turned to me and said, "I accept this." Her crying stopped immediately and from that point, my magnificent wife became a rock upon which all storms would surely break.

I, on the other hand, was in a state of shock, which isn't so bad; it sort of insulates and protects you from the initial impact. As the days passed, my shock slid into depression, so deep as to be blinding. Finally, the depression, too, began to wane, and that's when I was able to sit down and put everything into perspective.

My greatest fear and worry, and I don't think I'll ever get over this, is about my fourteen-month-old son and his at-risk status. If I knew he was safe and clear from this disease, I'd gladly offer myself up as the token sacrifice. But I don't know he will escape unscathed, and I can't seem to find peace when I think of my cherubic son. Instead, when I consider my son and his possible future, I just feel guilt, sorrow, and grief.

The possibility of HD being a reality to me was brought up just this last March. I had a conversation with a cousin whom I hadn't seen since we were kids. She told me that there was a risk of my getting HD, along with my brother and two sisters. Until that time, I had been led to believe that HD had missed my father. He died in a car crash at the age of fifty-five on his way home from work. His mother had Huntington's, as well as two of my uncles. Another brother died before showing any symptoms and both of my aunts, now in their seventies, have not shown symptoms.

After my conversation with my cousin, I went on the Internet and there, finally, read the reality of my situation as an at-risk person. The information I learned prompted me to look into testing, if not for myself, then for my wife and son.

I am able to begin to accept my situation with the help of my family. My mother has particularly been helpful as she instills in me a grain of hope, and each day that passes, that hope seems to take root further and help stabilize me. I find that I'm happy that I know what's in store for me, as opposed to having that void of knowledge. Knowledge is indeed strength, as it helps us to find things that bring peace and acceptance. It is my belief that if I can accept HD one hundred percent without fear or anger, then when Dr. Huntington does come knocking upon my door, this will be for the better. Maybe, just maybe, I will not exhibit the psychotic behavior to an extreme because I am not fighting or denying it and am instead accepting it.

I know that hope is a key ingredient to my present state of mind; hope that I have faith and hope that something good will come of this situation. I was agnostic before receiving my results, now I find I want God to exist more than anything else in the world. I want my prayers to be answered. I want God.

Huntington's Disease, for me, still represents oblivion. With each day that passes, I am speeding closer and closer into the arms of Dr. Huntington. I want to be able to look him in the eye and smile when I get to him, maybe even give him a hug and tell him he's not such a bad guy after all.

Why Me?

BY CARMEN LEAL-POCK

I gaze at the serene blue waters and wonder, "Why me?"
I ponder my shattered hopes and dreams and wonder,
   "Why me?"
I recall happier times, and wonder, "Why me?"

Sitting on the barren beach with waves splashing
   against the shore,
I feel as empty as the horizon.
As a lone tear drips off my chin and splashes onto the rocks,
I believe I can fill the ocean with the tears I have shed.
When my turbulent emotions become placid,
I think of my beautiful sons and wonder, "Why me?"
I reflect on my health, my family and friends and wonder,
   "Why me?"
I am blessed by thoughts of my church and wonder,
   "Why me?"

My mind fairly races with the joys of my life
I have somehow forgotten in my self-pity.
I consider a God so great He sent His Son to die
   on the cross for me,
and I wonder, "Why me?"
I am grateful that as Jesus hung on the cross
He didn't say, "Why me?"

An Answer to Prayer
BY CARMEN LEAL-POCK

It started with the simple household chores. Folding the laundry, washing dishes, cleaning a toilet or even screwing in a light bulb seemed beyond his ability. It wasn't that he lacked the willingness to help, he simply did an awful job of each chore. I refolded towels, restacked dishes and reswept floors, wondering what in the world was going on.

It would have been easier to understand if he had simply refused to help. But with his sweet smile and willing spirit, getting angry seemed counterproductive. It was easier to do all the chores myself than to be exasperated by his sloppy work.

I tried not to be unhappy with my choice of a husband, but little by little I felt the small seed of doubt creep in. Maybe I should have remained single. It wasn't that I didn't love him or enjoy his company. No, he was a wonderful husband and friend; there were just so many irritating things about him.

It seemed he could not drive without dinging or scraping the car. When he went to the store he inevitably brought home the wrong item. He spent money on foolish articles and bounced checks. This did not seem like the solid, sensible man I had married. From the beginning, my husband was always there with a helping hand for anyone who needed it. Was someone moving? Call Dave to help with the chore. Do the chairs need stacking at church? No problem, Dave will do it. There were not many constants in life, but one thing was sure; Dave would always help.

I continued my frantic pace of working outside the home and then rushing home to accomplish everything there. As my resentment grew, his energy waned. Little by little, all he seemed to do was sit in front of the television waiting to eat, finally to collapse for the eight or ten hours needed to recharge his batteries. I began to silently seethe inside and wonder what had changed my husband.

With the diagnosis of Huntington's Disease, I grasped the reason why; I saw the need to lower my expectations of what he could do each day. Though he would still help out if asked, I demanded less and less of him; the results of his labor only tended to produce a combination of depression and fury. In my head, I understood, yet the growing seeds of discontent had taken hold and were beginning to flourish.

I caught the sharp words of rebuke after they slipped from my lips. I was immediately sorry, but as my kids so often say, "Sorry doesn't help." I listened to my heavy sighs of exasperation and found myself rolling my eyes in disgust. Each time, my unkindness filled me with remorse and shame. He was dying, for goodness' sake! I was alive and vital. Why couldn't I just be kind and accept his growing deterioration instead of constantly criticizing him?

One day I began to pray, not for healing for David but for healing in myself. As my prayer began to unfold, it dawned on me that we are all terminal; what we can each do in the physical sense is gradually being diminished. I also knew that in response to his ebbing physical abilities, my spiritual gifts should be growing. The fact that in and of myself I could not stop being annoyed or disappointed struck me; only through Christ could I daily see value in my husband. I pleaded with God to help me accept David and his inabilities. I also prayed that He would grow me to the point that I could rejoice in the victories, no matter how minor they seemed.

One morning, I struggled out of bed to begin the day's frenzied pace still exhausted from an interrupted sleep; the thought of having to do everything myself was enough to drive me over the edge. Closing my eyes, I appealed to God. "Please, Lord. Give me just one reason to rejoice in my husband. Show me just one thing I don't have to do."

I dragged myself into the shower where the sharp spray would relax my aching body. I reached for the soap, and paused in thought. There are two things I can't stand. One is finding only a sliver of soap once I am wet, the second is finding no toilet paper when I need it. I stood amazed in the shower realizing God had answered my prayer. I had asked for just one thing that David could still do. In an instant, God had shown me two.

In the three years we have been married, I have never replaced the liquid or bar soap or the toilet tissue. I have taken for granted that they are always there when I need them. As much as David can't do, there are things he can do. God, knowing my irritations, made provisions for them by giving me a husband who has replaced innumerable rolls and soap bars. God's answer to that one small prayer made me realize that no matter how difficult life becomes, if I call out to Him, He will be gracious and answer me and comfort me in just the right way.

A Remembrance of Wayne
(FOR MY BUDDY, WHOM I NEVER MET)
BY HAROLD

It is Thursday
11:00 o'clock on a drizzly morning...
The Obit. column in the paper stated simply
And without any interpretation or significance:
Wayne... age fifty passed away Aug. 31st
At the city hospital,
And that the funeral would be today.

The cryptic announcement
Has no way of telling
About the heart-ache and grief...
The hopelessness of being helpless;
No way of explaining to people about
Those agonizing fifteen years
Of being completely dependent on others.

Perhaps there were some times when
The closest family members, in love, lost patience.
And the neurologists and doctors
Tried one cure after another...
Never to succeed in stopping
The terrible shaking and biting,
(Because of the disease we have named after Dr. Huntington).

Our mothers both had this sickness, Wayne.
Mine thought it was her change,
Until diagnosed correctly at a clinic.
We know now that her father, my grandfather
Prayed long agonizing hours on his knees

For God to take away his frightful temper and shaking;
He thought the devil was possessing him!

In our family the nerve deterioration
Comes some years later than in yours,
And I feel very deeply humbled...
Grateful that I still have some days
Of usefulness; but the agony
Of seeing your family suffer
Is very great.

Four years ago they took away
My driver's license. My feet were
Too shaky, I was an unsafe driver.
Foolishly I let this depress me,
Retreating more and more into myself.

But I don't dare look inward...
There is much yet to be done.
If God gives me more years, I am fifty-two
(Nearly the same as you.)
They must be spent in usefulness.
There is much yet to learn,
Of so many friendships and kindnesses.
There is comfort and uplift
At the Throne of God.
And for your family, today
Which is taking up its cross of suffering
You know that the Lord is already there,
To uphold you all and gird your feet
With a new strength.

In King David's life there were many joys,
And also heart-breaks.

His words from the 31st Psalm are:
"Be of good courage
And He shall strengthen your heart,
All ye that hope
In the Lord."

Rainy days and funerals... together they're depressing.
But when the rains stop
And the clouds move away
There is a burst of new sunshine
Cascading over our souls...
Reminding us that in all things,
We can fit within the Eternal Love and Plan of God.

ᦁ 13

Trisha's Story

BY TRISHA GAUGHAN

I MET Tom in December, 1989, just shortly after I moved from Washington State to Massachusetts. I was straight out of college and ready to begin my new life. Tom had a few odd facial movements, but I thought nothing of it. We went out a few times, and I remember saying, "I just want to be friends." Of course, the best plans often go awry, and somehow, he changed my heart. Tom is a tremendously loving, caring, and giving person. He is a special man not just to me, but to everyone he meets. When we were dating, he would send me cards. Do you know how hard it is to get a guy to send a card? But my Tom would sometimes send three or four cards a week. He used to carry around note cards with his name, address, and phone number on them and give them out to new friends. Yes, Tom was, and is, an incredible man. At one point in his life, his girlfriend at the time was going through trials as her father had lost his job. Tom wanted to give that family his whole paycheck. Common sense prevailed, but not many people would have considered doing that.

The thought of just being just friends with this man quickly left my mind, and on September 14, 1991, we were married. On this wonderful day, considering all the stress he was under, his movements were quite calm. Looking back, deep in my heart, I knew then that Tom had HD. Though I had never met his father, Tom Sr., I knew that he had died several years earlier from complications relating to HD. I didn't know anything about HD, so I once searched for information in a store Tom and I visited, but all I found was one little paragraph.

We settled happily into our newly married lives, until one day in October of 1991, Tom fainted. The emergency room doctor felt it was totally unrelated to HD, but he took me aside and recommended that we see a neurologist.

Tom and I had talked about this before and had decided that we would wait until we had kids before learning if Tom had Huntington's. After the emergency room visit, we decided to find a neurologist immediately. We visited the doctor at University Hospital who had seen Tom's father years earlier. At our first consult, the doctor sat down and said, "So, you have Huntington's Disease."

I was totally floored. There was no gentle easing into the conversation at all. After some additional talking he said, "I am going to diagnose you today." I cried in the office and Tom cried on the way home.

As much as I had known that he probably had HD, it was still a shock in the way it was presented. We had been married just a month and now everything was changing. We both stayed home for the next two and a half days and cried. We were sent for some tests, including an MRI, an EKG, and a neuro-psych, which all pointed to HD. After a follow-up visit, he wanted to send us for another test. We decided that we would look for a new doctor and so we declined the test and found Dr. Anne Young, whom we have been seeing ever since.

After much discussion, we knew two things. One, we still wanted children, and two we didn't want to run the risk of passing on this dreadful disease. Finally, in April of 1993, we visited Boston IVF (in-vitro fertilization). In July, 1993, during our second month of trying, we conceived a little boy by way of artificial insemination, using donor sperm. At this clinic, we gave the doctor a list of Tom's physical characteristics; the doctor chose the donor. It just seemed to work well this way, since I was not interested in making the decision.

People talk about the fact that they are willing to risk having a child because there is a fifty percent chance their baby won't have Huntington's Disease. That's true... but there is a fifty percent chance they will have it, too, and that was a risk we were not willing to take. Despite both of our desires to have Tom father this baby, I felt in my heart that our child would have HD. Tom's first symptoms appeared in his mid-twenties, and I realized with all I had learned that meant our child would probably become symptomatic even earlier.

Artificial insemination is a relatively simple procedure. The whole procedure takes about one minute, and is similar to the annual exam most women go through each year. The sperm is frozen and tested for AIDS, then after six months, a thorough family history is taken from the family. Now that I have my son, I can say I would not have done it any other way. Thomas III, named after his father and deceased grandfather, is such a delight; we are planning to do it again.

There is currently no cure for HD, but there is a way to stop the number of lives affected... by not passing on the gene. With all the scientific and medical advances, there are many alternative ways now available to have children. I recently watched a TV special where a man who has HD had twins with his sperm that are reported to be HD free. That was done using in-vitro fertilization. When there are eight cells in the embryo, one is removed and the genes are reviewed. Only the embryos that are free from HD are implanted into the woman.

This is just my story and how we dealt with a difficult situation. Morally, I struggled with my decision for quite some time. A missionary who was staying with us for a few days said, "Mary was artificially inseminated." While that may be a stretch, it put my mind at ease. The Bible did not give me clear guidance, but God put my heart at rest. Now I only look forward. I plan on telling my son as soon as he can understand, and I hope that someday I can meet the donor; I'm just naturally curious.

Shortly after Thomas was born, Tom, based on his own decision, chose to leave his job and apply for Social Security disability. Two weeks after we became parents, Tom had his last day at work; we both spent that summer at home. We had a wonderful time, filled with precious memories.

Tom is currently a full time daddy and we call him Mr. Mom. He says it is the best job he has ever had. For now, he does a great job caring for three-year-old Thomas. If Tom becomes unable to care for our son, I will place Thomas in daycare or find someone to come to the house. It works out well because Tom collects disability, and is Mr. Mom. He does all the laundry, loads and unloads the dishwasher, cleans the bathroom, looks after and plays with Thomas, and changes diapers. My mother-in-law lives only five minutes away and is there to help whenever either of us needs her, which is not often. I could not handle this disease without the help of my in-laws. They have said that they will help us when Tom gets sick and have already helped us in many little ways; they have taken Tom and Thomas to the doctor, watched Thomas a few times, and even took Thomas for twelve days while Tom and I traveled to England this year to celebrate my thirtieth birthday.

I cannot, and do not, go to work and worry about Thomas' safety. I find it impossible to function like that. But I do watch Tom's progression carefully and cater to both of their needs as best I can. Tom enjoys his role as Mr. Mom and likes being home. I truly believe the love and attention of Thomas has helped Tom to fight this disease. He remains completely functional, except work and driving, despite having the chorea for nearly ten years now. Tom believes that someday God will heal him completely so he can work and drive again. While I believe that God can heal Tom, I think that it is not probable. Thus, I plan for the worst as best I can.

One of the areas where more planning would have made sense is insurance. We were ignorant and did not get extra life insurance before seeing the neurologist. I do have a modest life insurance policy on Tom through my work, and he is also covered under my health insurance policy. I have switched policies and have not had a problem with his coverage. Along with social security disability, we receive a small amount each month from a disability policy from Tom's work.

I do have some concern about raising a child with a terminally ill parent, but I do know that children are strong. They adapt and you just have to extend yourself to help them grow up healthy. Thomas is not the only child ever born into a potentially adverse situation; many who have lived through worse have grown into healthy, happy adults. I wanted what everyone else had, selfish or not.

People who think that we shouldn't have kids are not in our shoes. It is easy for someone in a healthy, normal marriage with kids to say you shouldn't, but I could not imagine my life without kids. For now, Thomas is a loving, happy, joyous child. I will devote whatever resources, time, and attention I can to ensure he stays healthy, both mentally and emotionally. When the time is right, we will tell Thomas about his Daddy so it will not be a shock thrown at him when he is a teen.

Since I've known Tom, we have lived as if HD was not a part of our lives. We bought a house, we have a donor baby, and we take vacations. I have planned, as best I can, to protect our life. We put our house in a trust and have a fifteen-year mortgage, and I will extend it to thirty years when Tom is sick so I can reduce my work schedule. Of course, the goal is to pay the house off before that point.

We have built up quite a support system, and that too helps in looking towards the future. That system includes our friends Bill and B.B. They took Tom under their wing when Tom Sr. was hospitalized. He went on vacation with them, and was treated like one of their own children. Bill and B.B. continue to provide us with tremendous emotional support. We have many other friends who are really "family" to us, and we know they will give us strength and support whenever we need it. Tom's parents, Ed and Charlotte, have also been extremely supportive. They supported us in our decision to have children and help out however they can. When I need them, or others, I won't have to look far. I know that I am not in this thing alone.

I don't know how I will do everything, but I know that God will provide.

When Tom is at his worst, I hope to reduce my work schedule to two or three days a week, devoting my time to his care and attention. I plan on fighting to get home health aides and other home services. I will not have my son taking care of daddy. He will help, I'm sure, but he deserves as normal a life as possible, and that includes time for sports, music lessons, friends, vacations, and doing his best in school. Thomas will have his grandparents to help him through this as well, and he will have the opportunity to escape from HD through camp and flying to visit my parents in Washington State. If I can no longer provide the best care for Tom, I will arrange to send him to the Lowell-Mediplex Center in Lowell, Massachusetts. This is a well run home, with a compassionate administrator, that has a large number of HD patients.

For this one person, for this one family history, we stopped Huntington's Disease. This is my contribution to the ending of this terrible scourge. There are doctors and scientists around the world fighting to find a cure. We were not willing to wait for the cure, and now, no other Tom Gaughan's will have this beast of a disease. It will not continue to be passed on, knowingly or blindly, to our innocent children or grandchildren. I pray Thomas III will have a long, prosperous life. He may suffer through the hardships endured by his dad, but he and I will prevail with God's help. God is with us every minute of every day.

ᦂ 14

Faces of Forgiveness

BY CARMEN LEAL-POCK

I can forgive, but I cannot forget, is only another way of saying, I will not forgive. Forgiveness ought to be like a canceled note – torn in two, and burned up, so that it never can be shown against one.

—Henry Ward Beecher

There is so much that is painful about Huntington's; even to those who don't have the gene. The cruelty of the disease is compounded by the dynamics of things we have experienced in the past, and will experience in the future. In my situation, I had already gone through a marriage that had ended in turmoil. Meeting Dave, a man who cherished me as no one had before, filled me with hope for a future filled with happiness.

When Dave and I went through pre-marital counseling, I remember being asked about my greatest fear for this marriage. "Having to care for Dave when he gets old is my greatest fear," I said. "I don't do sick, and I want to die before Dave does so I won't have to care for him."

The second question I remember involved my expectations for the marriage. There were many, but some of them included the expectation of a partner for decades to come, someone to be a role model for my children, a handyman to fix my dilapidated house, and a partner to earn enough to make us comfortable. I didn't think any of those were unrealistic expectations.

When Dave was diagnosed three years into our marriage, I, of course, knew that my fears had been realized, and that my expectations would not be met. I was angry; not so much at Dave as with the disease and the circumstances. But what could I do but go on? And so we went on, finding solutions to problems and doing the best we could.

One solution involved uprooting my teenage sons and moving to a different state. It was hard, but I didn't see other options at the time. Knowing there was no nursing home in Hawaii that would take a person with HD, I realized I would probably move eventually, and it may as well be now. I was angry at having to pull my children away from the only home they had ever known, but we would adjust.

After six months of struggling to make a life for ourselves in Florida, Dave made a stunning announcement. One morning he woke up and told me he had a confession to make. "I knew I was sick when I asked you to marry me," he said.

"You knew you had Huntington's?" I gasped.

"No, I knew I was sick. I thought I had Multiple Sclerosis."

Dave's mother had been adopted, and when we married, she was living in another state in the final stages of what he thought was Multiple Sclerosis.

"I don't care what initials you put on it, MS or HD; it doesn't really matter, you lied to me," I yelled. How could he not tell me something of this magnitude, especially when I had told him my biggest fears, my greatest expectations? Our marriage had been a lie from day one, and I could never forgive him.

Dave depends on me to feed him and provide for most of his other needs. I told him, with contempt, that I had to sort things out in my mind and I could not be around him until I was ready. He would just have to starve, and with that I got out of bed and left the room. Of course, he didn't starve, and eventually I had a choice to make. Undeniably, what he had done was wrong. I didn't know if he had lied by omission because his mind was already severely affected, or because he was afraid of being alone. Maybe he lied because he loved me and feared my rejecting him. I had certainly given him every reason to believe I would not marry him, since I had told him how much I would hate caring for a sick person.

Over the next few weeks, I cared for Dave and was civil to him, but just barely. I spoke with a pastor at church, and cried out my anguish to my on-line support group. My ladies' bible study group also listened to my dilemma. I knew in my heart there was absolutely no way I would have married someone with a disease as crippling as MS, let alone one with even greater ramifications, like HD. I certainly would never have dragged my children into this mess that had caused me to lose all I had and continue to rack up piles of debt.

I received advice from many, and the vast majority were appalled at his disclosure, urging me to find a nursing home for him, get a divorce, and begin my life again. The temptation to do just that was never far from my mind. Our marriage had been built on lies, I argued with myself. I had no moral obligation to remain, provided I made sure he was taken care of. I found myself becoming more short-tempered with my children and more unhappy with myself as the battle within me raged.

Praying and asking God for direction one day, I thought of something that helped me forgive Dave. Previously, I had devised this exercise, including a section on forgiving for divorced or widowed people. In the group, after we had discussed forgiveness, we talked about how not only must we forgive, but we also must ask for forgiveness from our past spouses, who may or may not forgive us. In addition, we also need to seek God's forgiveness daily.

I knew that although I had not told Dave a lie about my health, there were areas of failure in our marriage on my part, too. I needed to ask Dave for forgiveness, as well as I needed to forgive him.

In the group, I passed out a piece of paper and told everyone to go home and write a letter to God, confessing their sins and asking for His forgiveness. They were to tell Him how much they had hurt Him and how sorry they were. And then tear up the letter and throw it aside. The next day they were to come back, pick up the letter and tape it together, writing more details of the sin, and making sure to embellish them wherever possible. They were to pray about the sins again, and ask for forgiveness; tear it up into smaller pieces and place it aside once more. I told the group to repeat the exercise as many times as they thought it takes for God to forgive them.

Even without doing the exercise myself, this time I knew the answer. God forgives us the first time we ask. We are the ones who persists in pulling our sins out of the trash over and over, piecing them together and making them look worse than we could ever imagine.

Not only does God forgive us, but He tells us to forgive, no matter how "bad" the sin. There is nothing I can do that God won't forgive me for the first time I ask Him. In my retelling of the situation, I had made it worse and worse in my mind. I had fashioned Dave into a liar of the worst type who had sought me out intentionally to destroy my life. Of course, that wasn't true at all. Dave was a desperately sick man, with a disease that had already begun to rob him of his ability to make right decisions. He made a mistake, but that did not mean he didn't deserve love and should be abandoned. I knew that if I chose to walk away, God would still love me and forgive me all my sins. But would that be the right thing to do? At that instant, I forgave Dave, and recommitted myself to give him the best care he deserved. And I accepted God's forgiveness for my sins, too.

There are so many aspects of Huntington's Disease that can destroy us if we let them. Each person dealing with this insidious disease has someone or something that has hurt them and devastated some part of their lives. The disease itself, the hidden knowledge of the family gene, someone treating you like a leper or being abandoned should make you angry. Anger is a very real part of life and needs to be dealt with. Eventually, though, the anger, if left unchecked, will act as a cancer to destroy relationships, and eventually, bodies, minds, and souls.

Jennifer James says, "Sometimes we find it hard to forgive. We forget that forgiveness is as much for us as for the other person. If you can't forgive it's like holding a hot coal in your hand.... you're the one getting burned. The tension may be hurting you much more than the other person."

It takes the act of forgiveness to heal what anger would destroy. We need to forgive others, but not only because they need our forgiveness; forgiving others releases us from the resentment, hostility, and rage we hold onto when we don't forgive them. To heal ourselves of the wounds inflicted upon us, we must be willing to forgive those who hurt us, totally and completely. Forgiveness makes us whole again.

∽

Apology
BY SHERRY LEE

"Research is needed to halt the progress of the illness in those who already carry the gene. But the destruction of HD is already available to all who know it is present; we don't have to pass it on! Let it die with the DNA of those who suffer from it, let that be the finest and most courageous sacrifice a pHD can make."

—Daleah Caprice Thiessen

I was an at-risk individual who, in my teen years, made decisions to have children early in life. By doing this, I thought, I would be free from Huntington's Disease long enough to raise them. I was educated in the genetics of the disease, but obviously not old enough to be realistic about what my children would have to live with. I now know it was a given that my children would be affected by HD. Whether living to take care of me, living only to inherit the disease themselves, or living with a parent who continually obsessed about if she had the disease, they would be affected.

It was, at the very least, an incredibly selfish decision. I was only thinking of myself. At eighteen, I already had two children, and was secure in my mind that I had made the right decision. I love my children more than life itself;

but as I grew older, the question of whether I had made the right decision haunted me. I would cry at night, watching them sleep, thinking, "How could I do this to them? What will life really be like for them ten years down the road?"

I knew first hand what it was like having a parent with HD. I had lived with my father's rages and unforgivable beatings. I had endured the staring from school mates when he committed suicide. Is this what I wanted for the people I loved? Did I make the right decisions? Can anyone really answer that?

I am a good mom. I wipe noses, and rock away bad dreams. I meet the teachers, and I pack the lunches. But if you asked my mother when the parenting stops, she would surely say that it never does. At twenty-eight, I need to call her and ask for wisdom. I feel robbed of the father that I should have had; he wasn't there to give me away at my wedding. I didn't have a father to be proud of me, or mad at me. What made me think that my children would need me any less than I needed, still need, my father? Even by having them so young, did I really ensure that they would be OK if I did have HD?

When I went through the predictive testing a year ago, my worst fear was that my husband would leave me, and my children would despise me. I hated wondering if I had destroyed my children's lives. I truly regretted my decision to have them, even if I did love them. It seemed like abuse to me that I would willfully let them live with the fear of this monster. I had thought of leaving them all, to run away like a child some place else. I would just live alone. And die alone. But it wouldn't erase what they would inevitably have to face themselves. Had I made the right decisions? Yes and no. I escaped it because I tested negative. It took almost a month to stop crying. I could look at my children and breathe for the first time in years. If I had to live my life over, would I have had them? Probably. I am selfish, I will admit that, and I love my children. I love them with the kind of love that is hard to give up. But I do owe them an apology. I should have cared enough to think of them completely before I had them.

∼

Till Death Do Us Part
BY RUTH HARGRAVE

Life has not gone the way I dreamed it would in 1952 when Bill and I married, but it has been infinitely more exciting than I imagined. Bill and I were childhood sweethearts, having dated all four years of his navy service and my high school days. I had just graduated and Bill was discharged after serving his country for four years. As I waited at the aisle for him to make me his bride, I knew there was no one more handsome than this tall, lean man in uniform. What could possibly go wrong to mar the perfection of that day?

Within five years, I was the mother of four adorable children; two boys and two girls. Besides the busy times brought on by motherhood, I helped Bill in the business. We were occupied in building a trailer court in upstate New York, and that meant we did all the physical labor. One time we laid a sewer pipe during a snow storm and ended up laughing with a foot of snow on our backs from bending over digging. As hard as it was, we didn't mind; it was a labor of togetherness.

As the years marched on, the children grew and my family moved to Virginia Beach, VA. We decided to follow suit, selling the business and moving there to my mother's trailer court. The area's work force was either the navy or

Norfolk Southern Railroad, and since Bill no longer wanted to be a navy man, he donned a railroad conductor's hat and began his third and final career. Then in 1984, he fell from the top of a moving railroad car and lost both legs.

Bill had always been a heavy drinker and his time in the hospital was rough. He was in the trauma unit for three months and on the regular floor for another month. After he came home, strange things would happen; his hands would fly all over and he had trouble sitting on the commode; he would yell out in the middle night. His behavior got uglier every day. After thirty-five years of marriage, it seemed I couldn't please him in any way. At first, I thought it was the loss of his legs and the withdrawal from all the medication he had been receiving. At that point, he was so violent, and his behavior so increasingly weird, I had him committed. This man, whom I had loved most of my life, seemed to be gone and a monster had taken his place.

After the doctor at the hospital saw Bill bite the nurse, he suggested that perhaps Bill had Huntington's Disease. I had never heard of that before in his family, nor had his mother who was still going strong at eighty-five; he knew of no one in her family with this disease. Bill's father had died at age thirty-five in a motorcycle accident, his grandmother died of alcoholism and his great-grandmother committed suicide. Still, I said to myself, I was not going to believe Huntington's was the problem until I could see some proof.

When the doctors prescribed Haldol and Prozac, he changed overnight. Yes, it did dope him in the beginning, but that was a relief for me. He stayed on that dosage and as time went by, he got used to it and seemed somewhat normal. The drugs arrested his movements; that was even more important than with most HD sufferers because he had no legs.

Eventually, our third child began having what seemed liked HD symptoms. It took three years before she was able to seek help at Johns Hopkins. The DNA test was performed on her and on our second child, who had by that time also become symptomatic. Following their positive results, we sent Bill's blood in and, of course, at long last, the diagnosis became a reality. All three of them had HD.

I went to the library for information, but there was very little available. Until my husband died in 1995, I just stumbled through caring for him the best I knew. It was hard because by then we had a house and twelve acres; I had to deal with well water and pumps and lawn mowers that didn't start – and become an auto mechanic. It was necessary because we lived in a rural area. We even had a wood stove to help heat the house, and I had the cutest little chain saw. I would take the cutting deck off the lawn and garden tractor, and go into the woods dragging down a small fallen tree, which I then cut up. My husband would wheel his chair up to the window and watch with a smile on his face. He didn't talk much, and I often wondered what was going on behind those large brown eyes of his.

After the accident, I took over the household bill paying. It was then that I noticed numerous long distance phone calls to upstate New York. That was the beginning of finding out that my husband had had an affair while we were living in upstate New York. He was now phoning this woman after many years of no contact with her. The affair was back in 1956 and I didn't find out until thirty years later; all those years. To say I was crushed and angry is an understatement. This was not the way it was supposed to be. My husband was my Prince Charming, so where was our happily ever after? Instead of living a storybook life, I was trapped in a marriage to a legless monster who supposedly had some disease I knew nothing about. I later found out that not only had he had the affair, but a child had been born from that union and had the possibility of having the disease. And if she had Huntington's, any of her children had a fifty percent chance of getting it, too. How could I ever begin to have whatever it would take to be his caregiver and forgive him?

Helmut Thielicke, a German pastor who endured horrors at the hands of the Nazi Third Reich, is quoted as saying, "Forgiveness does not mean that we will forget. No, we remember, but in forgiving we no longer use the memory against others, or ourselves. Forgiveness is not pretending that the offense did not really matter. It did matter and it does matter, and there is no use pretending otherwise. The offense is real, but when we forgive, the offense no longer controls our behavior or emotions. Forgiveness is not acting as if things are just the same as before the offense. We face the fact that things will never again be the same, but, by the grace of God, they can be better...."

I now know that inappropriate sexual behavior is often one of the hallmarks of Huntington's Disease. Bill had been symptomatic for years and his behavior was really a product of the disease, not a desire to destroy our marriage. I realized that the person who would be hurt the most by my lack of forgiveness was me; I would be eaten inside like a cancer and turn into a bitter, hateful woman. Even if Bill didn't think he needed me, my children did.

I was dealing with his infidelity and caring for him, all the while knowing what my children would be facing. It was a painful time, but somehow God knew what I needed to get me through that period of my life. I am a painter and a lover of art. Looking back, my best work was produced while under tremendous stress. When my husband died, I focused on my daughter. She had two children by this time, and though the oldest was on her own, her young son still needed care. My son-in-law was long gone, so I decided to take the money that I had and build an addition to my home. This addition would be a place for my HD positive son, daughter and at-risk grandson. It was a huge expense, but at that point, these two adult children of mine had no one but me. The Lord had entrusted them to me; like this was my destiny to care for them.

Living in a situation like this is not easy. At sixty-four years of age, I am trying to raise a fifteen-year-old while dealing with all sorts of challenges, including suicide attempts, alcoholism, and mood swings. My plate is full, but if the truth be known, I have the privilege of knowing my children more deeply than most parents. We share a lot, living in the same house.

Bill's last gift to us was the donation of his brain to Johns Hopkins research. It might be his tissue that breaks through a cure for us all. Life rarely plays out the way we anticipate, but it does play out the way God wants it to. And that's all that really matters.

∽

Always on My Mind
BY MARY CHRISTOPHER

As I write this, it will be twenty-five years tomorrow, March 29th, that Elvis first recorded this song... about a month before his separation from Priscilla. Most people, on hearing the song and knowing that Elvis' marriage was on the rocks, believe that Elvis had Priscilla in mind when he sang the song. It is this which gives the song such authenticity and depth, and one cannot help but be moved by it, especially when also seeing Elvis' facial expression on video as he sings it.

I have another story to tell about the song, one with a happy ending.

I am writing a book, a section of which reports how the songs Elvis sang have affected people spiritually. I have been asking fans to relate to me their stories of how a particular song has brought encouragement, hope and healing, and have heard some very interesting and moving stories. This one occurred recently and involves myself.

We have three wonderful children, now all adults. Recently, on a weekend visit, our younger daughter, now twenty years old, suddenly confided in me that as a teenager she had felt very insecure and not good enough. This surprised me; she is, and always has been very outgoing and vivacious. I was also taken aback, because we have always thought of our family as being very close and loving, and yet I had not noticed my daughter's unhappiness in those years. A few days later, I was led to carefully listen to the words of 'Always on My Mind,' sung by Elvis. While listening, I shed many tears, mostly of regret, that I hadn't always treated her as good as I should have, that I didn't take the time to tell her that I am so happy that she is my daughter, or hold her in all those lonely, lonely times. I was so sorry that I was blind and made her feel second best.

Having shed the tears and feeling a release, I then wrote out the words of the song and sent them to our daughter, with a note saying that was how I felt about our relationship, and that she was and always will be on my heart and mind.

The wonderful result is that, although we were close, a barrier has been broken down and our relationship has changed. We are so much closer, and will always be able to confide in each other and keep our relationship full of love and commitment. I want to thank the songwriters Carson,

James and Christopher for the powerful words of the song, Elvis for the powerful singing of the song, but most of all, Jesus Christ for the power of forgiveness. I would encourage anyone who has someone, who has a wife, husband, mother, father, brother, sister, daughter, son, friend, neighbor, colleague, to regularly inspect their relationship with the words of this song in mind; then, if there are any causes of regret, to share them with the person, and stand back and watch the healing take place!

$\backsim$

This Man Was Me
BY SHIRLEY PROCELL

As I wandered through this land
I met a man I could not stand
He stared at me with soulful eyes
And then I came to realize
That I must walk this land again
Take this person, as my friend
For after looking close, you see
I found this man was really me
I did not like what I'd become
Or many things that I had done
First I needed to forgive
Forget, and change the way I lived
To see the good in someone else
You, first, must learn to like yourself
So when I walk this land again
I might become my own best friend.

15

Tom's Story

BY TOM GILLIHAN

HELEN and I first met in the spring of 1975 when we were eighteen and sixteen. Mature for her age, she was very pretty, and, like me, quiet and shy. From the first time we met, we just seemed to fit together well. Helen lived alone with her mom and had four older brothers already on their own.

She didn't talk much about her dad, only that her mom and dad had been divorced since she was little, both had remarried and her mom eventually divorced again. Later that year, I found out that her dad was in a mental hospital in Portland, Oregon, and had something called Huntington's Chorea. I felt badly about her dad, but since I had never heard of that disease, I didn't think it would affect us.

In December of that year, Helen got information from the University of Washington about some research being done on persons with a connection to HD. They requested that she go to the university for some tests. I took her, and they did some basic reflex tests; they found nothing unusual. They also told us more about the disease and her chances of getting it. That was a little scary, but we were young and indestructible. We talked about it, deciding to go ahead and marry, partly because we were in love, and partly because Helen could no longer live with her mom. Not knowing Helen's fate, we were married on March 27, 1976.

We talked about the risks of having kids and decided all of life is a risk. Even if Helen did get HD, the chances were good that they would find a cure by the time our children were old enough to get it. Besides, Helen's dad was sixty years old now, so we figured Helen had at least thirty years before she would even have to worry about it.

Our first son was born in April of the following year and his brother came along in November of 1978. Things went along great for a few years. We never talked about HD or Helen's dad. It was as if the possibility of our happiness being dimmed by this dreadful sickness did not exist.

A couple of years later, we found out that one of Helen's brothers had it. He was thirty-four or thirty-five at the time. We couldn't believe how quickly he went downhill. We hadn't seen him in a few years and it was alarming to see him now; this was the first time I had seen anyone affected by HD. Afterwards, Helen told me that if she did get this disease, she would kill herself. In August of 1982, we got news that Helen's dad was dying, so we went to the mental hospital to see him. I swore then that I would never let Helen go to a place like that if I could prevent it.

The next April, her brother with HD died at thirty-eight. Tragically, one of her other brothers died in a car wreck on the way to the funeral. This was a terrible time for Helen, but we still didn't talk about the possibility of her getting it. Instead, we talked about our future together, all the things we were going to do, and places we would go as soon as the kids were out on their own. We shared our dreams of all the places we wanted to visit in our travels and about retirement and growing old together.

However, all our plans for the future were not enough to make a difference. Gradually, I could see changes; she became moody, got upset over little things. As the new decade became a reality, she began to drop things repeatedly. We had always gone for daily walks of two or three miles, time and weather permitting. But now Helen started slowing down on those walks. It was getting harder for her to walk any distance, and we cut our walks to one mile, often even less. She just didn't seem to have any energy even for something so simple as walking.

In the summer of 1994, we decided to check into the testing for HD. Helen was having more problems, but she was still convinced that she did not have HD. We went to a genetic counselor, then to a neurologist where they wanted her to have a CT scan (computerized tomography), which is an advanced X-ray technique showing detailed cross sections of the brain. At that point, she changed her mind and didn't go any further. A year later, when she started having severe pain in her lower leg muscles, we went back to the neurologist and then had the CT scan. By this time, the progression of the disease was far enough along that the CT scan showed clear signs of HD. It was almost a relief to know for sure that it was HD causing all the problems and not something else. But this was also the end to our distant future together. Now we only talked about what we would do the next day, or the next week, but not the next year. Because we didn't know if there would be a next year.

Sometimes I would think about the future alone and wonder, "How long will Helen be around." I thought about whether I could go on alone after being married for so long, and wondered how I would take care of her, the kids, the house and a full time job.

The following year, Helen deteriorated at a rapid pace. She talked about trying to kill herself several times and even tried once. By March of 1996, she needed a wheelchair to go shopping or out for walks. She could still walk, but was falling a lot. In April, we started having nursing aides come to the house to help a couple of hours a day, to help with meals and medication while I was at work. By July, she could no longer stay by herself at all; it was just too dangerous. At that point, we began having aides there the whole time I was at work. Her moods were swinging drastically from minute to minute sometimes and it was like living on a roller coaster all the time. You never knew what might set her off. The boys and I walked on egg shells constantly, trying to keep her calm.

Then in the middle of August, she went off the deep end. I came home one evening to find her so worked up that she was totally soaked with sweat. Like a woman possessed, she was throwing her body around violently and screaming that she wanted to die and asking me to help her kill herself. It was one of the worst moments of my life. One part of me would have liked to help her end the suffering, but the rest of me didn't want to lose her. I tried for a couple of hours to calm her down, with no luck. I finally gave up and took her to the emergency room at the hospital where they checked her into the mental ward where she stayed for a week. They changed her medications before she came home. In September, she started hallucinating badly. Every day she would tell me how terrible the aides were to her, how they were trying to kill her and how other people were after her. When she decided she wanted to go to a nursing home, I tried to talk her out of it and so did the doctor. But she was convinced that only there would she be safe. With resignation, we visited a few of them around town until she picked the one she wanted. She was admitted in early October, 1996.

It was difficult trying to educate the staff and aides about HD, but they worked hard and have done a good job... considering most of them had never heard of this disease before meeting Helen. The hard part for me, personally, was just the idea of no longer being able to take care of my loving wife of twenty years. Helen was now only thirty-seven years old; I felt I had somehow let her down.

That first day in the home will always stick in my mind. She looked so out of place there. Here she was, still so young, living with all these old people who were waiting to die. When I left that first day, I went out to my car and just sat and cried. I couldn't believe I had really done this to her. When I got home, the house felt so empty and alone without her there. If it weren't for my kids still at home, now seventeen and nineteen, and the on-line support group, I don't think I would have made it.

The kids seem to take all this in stride and go about their own lives. I try to talk to them occasionally about the whole thing with their mom; that they are at risk of ending up the same way. They are young and don't seem to have time to worry or even think about it, so I just try to leave the subject open for when they do have time.

Helen has done pretty well in the home. She has been there almost a year now, and I spend as much time as possible with her, usually four or five hours a day. It is still very hard for me to leave her some days. It's a roller coaster ride, with good days and bad, but we try to always take one day at a time. One especially tough part of this disease is the frustrations of Helen's decreasing communication skills. Some days I can understand everything she says, and other days, after having her repeat herself for the third or fourth time, we both get frustrated and give up. I know it is very hard on her when she wants something and can't get anyone to understand what it is. But it is just as hard for me when all I want to do is please her, and I can't figure out what she wants.

I think the hardest part of the disease for me to deal with are the mental problems. I can compensate for most of the physical losses, but the mental ones I can't do anything about. The only way I can cope is to go back to taking one day at a time. Sometimes, on good days, I can still look into her eyes and see the beautiful young girl I married, and it keeps me going back another day. I still love her now as much as I did twenty-two years ago, maybe more.

Some nights I lay in bed looking at the empty place beside me, and wish things could be the way they once were... but I know that they won't. There are days when I awake in the morning feeling sorry for myself, trying to find a reason to get up. Then I think of her, and all she's going through, and the knowledge of her waiting for me to get there and how lonely she must feel. Then I feel ashamed of my self-pity, so I get up and start another day.

On August 12, 1997, shortly after Tom told his story, his beautiful wife Helen passed away in the nursing home.

For Helen

SHIRLEY PROCELL

HD claimed another
Yes, an Angel is gone
Taken by the Father
To her heavenly Home
Let us not weep
Or very long, mourn
This Angel's body
Has just been reborn
She's in a place
Where pain is unknown
Right beside God
As he sits on his throne
Someday we will join her
As our lives here end
Join her in Heaven
For real life to begin.

Written in memory of Helen Gillihan , sadly missed by her family and her extended family, here on Hunt-Dis.

~ 16

Faces of Hope

BY CARMEN LEAL-POCK

I do not want to look back and say, "I wish we had..." but be able to say, " I am so glad we did." And when that miracle happens and a cure is found, well I can say, "Let's just do it again!"

—Mary Jean McGee

Today, while driving on my round of errands, I listened to a radio station where songs of romance dominate. Love in first bloom to love on the rocks are common themes, equally popular heard from male and female vocalists. One song I heard was particularly moving. It spoke, at the time, about grief and pain.

In his song, "Tears In Heaven," Eric Clapton has written a powerful message about death and those left behind. Although touched by the ballad from the first moment I heard it, I have to admit surprise that the jaded entertainment industry awarded Clapton his greatest fame ever for a song about death. At the Grammy Awards, "Tears in

Heaven" received the Grammy as the "Song of the Year." The album that contained it won "Album of the Year," and Mr. Clapton himself was applauded as "Male Vocalist of the Year."

Fans around the world grieved with the family when it was learned that the singer's four-year-old son had fallen to his death from a fifty-third floor New York city apartment building. In a few moving moments, Clapton acknowledges that death, sings of the assurance that his son is in heaven, and admits his grief and the need to be strong. Although the song is obviously filled with despair, the chorus affirms that there is hope. This tribute, with the haunting refrain, offers us a ray of sunshine when it insists there will be no tears in heaven.

Clapton would love to rest in heaven with his son, but he knows it is not yet his time and he will have to carry his own sorrow. The hope that he sings of is in the future for himself, and the present for his little boy.

That Eric Clapton won such acclaim for that song is a testament not only to his thirty years as an entertainer, but to our need to find hope in the midst of such tragedy. As people who are currently in the thick of the battle, we all have moments of true grief. No one can deny the heartbreak when the diagnosis of Huntington's is confirmed. As we daily watch our loved ones become more incapacitated, our hearts cry out at the cruelty of this disease. Even those whose tests return negative don't escape the overwhelming sadness that accompanies loss. An at-risk status indicates an HD parent, and that in itself implies grief in the past, present or in the future.

I have heard people in HD circles say that they would prefer having cancer as an opponent. With cancer and other illnesses, there is still hope. Chemotherapy, surgery, radiation and other aggressive therapies all offer hope in otherwise seemingly hopeless situations. For those of us touched by Huntington's, however, there is no immediate medical hope. Oh, there are ways to manage some of the symptoms... but that's all. How, then, can one say there are faces of hope?

Hope comes in many packages and can be vastly different for each of us. The hope Eric Clapton expressed in his son's happiness in heaven gave him a reason to live. This is a common expression of hope at funerals and memorial services. We all hope and pray for a cure and we know great strides are being made in that direction. Others hope for negative results in their testing or in that of their children.

I believe that even while some people express a total lack of faith, they do have some hope, fleeting as it may be. A young woman, who has questioned her own hope told me of this experience. She said that her young man, for lack of a better term, is gene-positive. They've broken up once already over his gene status because he's afraid of hurting her once he becomes symptomatic, among other reasons. They're back together now, or at least as together as two people can be when separated by three thousand miles. They are both twenty-four, neither of them is religious and she does not have a belief in God. After being on this support list, reading message after message about prayers and faith and putting one's trust in God, she wonders where it leaves her. She feels alienated from the list, and especially hopeless, since so many people have said that God is the chief way they get through life with Huntington's. She doesn't know where to find hope since she supposes she doesn't really have much... beyond her blind, arrogant, twenty-four-year-old assurance that both of them will live forever. This statement she made says so much. "So, no, I guess I don't have a lot of hope. What I do have is a heart full of worry, a gut full of helpless rage and a jaw-grinding determination to just keep going, whatever the end."

Even in her statement of hopelessness, we see hope. She has hope in herself that she will get through this. Sometimes that is all people do have; hope in themselves.

Jim, a friend from the on-line support group, also finds hope... but not in a place connected to his faith or God.

"It is really difficult to find hope after eleven years of fighting HD. Where is the hope when a healthy, robust father of two, or three or four, becomes a shaking, violent opposite of what he has been for all his life? It is really difficult to find hope when the woman you hoped to live your silver and golden years with is unable to walk and blames you for the disease she has been given.

"Despite all of this," he continues, "I guess I get the most hope from this mailing list. I am encouraged when I read about how the different techniques have helped those we love overcome various problems. I learn how different medications help diminish some of the symptoms, and how the fetal cell program is doing, and I find hope. I get hope from friends with words of encouragement and help. I get hope from the younger people on the list who struggle with the decision to test or not, and the reasons they give for their decisions. Those that have been struggling with this disease for so long and have not given up fill me with hope. Hope is in the information shared by the professionals and in the dedicated researchers that are working to find a treatment, and eventually a cure for this horrible disease." Jim goes on to say, "I guess the list is the only place that I really get any hope at all, and it is the most important and useful place for me."

For others, Hope is entwined in their faith. This is Sue Powell's story.

"I will tell you where the hope I have comes from; the Lord. My dad has HD and I know that the love he has for God is what he leans on for strength and peace. When we found out about my dad and Huntington's over a year ago, and I realized that I was at-risk for this horrid disease, I have to say that my emotional state of mind was anything but peaceful. I went through what I can only describe as grieving. Grieving for what it meant for my dad, what it could mean for me, and worst of all, what it might mean for my children. It was a rough time for me. I kept reaching out to Jesus for help, and guess what? He gave it! One day as I was praying and crying out to God, asking Him why, I felt His presence and His love surround me. It was as if He was standing right there hugging me! I realized at that moment that I had nothing to fear because He would always be there, for me, for my dad and also for my children." Sue is emphatic. She says, "I can get through anything in this world, including HD, as long as God is by my side. Do I still get scared sometimes? Yes. Do I still cry when I see my dad being taken over by the debilitation of HD? Yes. Do I still get sad thinking about my kids? Yes. Do I believe that the good Lord can provide peace and joy and happiness in the midst of and despite all this? Yes! He is my hope. It is hard to sum up and put into mere words the bounds of this love that God has for those who accept and believe in Him. It is powerful and empowering and it provides the peace that surpasses all understanding."

I have met others, who are so filled with despair, that they sabotage relationships so others won't be hurt when they become symptomatic. They are anything but hopeful. Huntington's Disease has one of the highest suicide rates of any terminal disease. That tells us some people cannot find hope in anything but a release from the inevitable.

Hope can be found in the love we share with our families and friends, the joy in life outside HD and, of course, the hope that exists through our faith. But sometimes hope is ill-founded. That can be the basis of a disaster.

Shortly after college, I joined the Peace Corps. I was assigned to one of the poorest countries in the world. Living in Mali, West Africa, I taught English as a foreign language to high school students. My first year was spent in the capital, but the second year was spent in the Sahara Desert in the city of Gao. Mali is landlocked with no resources of its own. As such, it has remained relatively unexploited. Although Mali is definitely an underdeveloped country, my desert home boasted all the creature comforts, including mud construction, an indoor bathroom, and running water. Of course, only the first was guaranteed, since we had water for just thirty minutes daily, usually at 4:00 a.m.

Life in a country where one has to speak more than one foreign language was hard. Considering that I taught several classes of sixty students, bargained for food, chopped wood and killed chickens, there were days when I had very little hope of finishing my two years. One day, I had a friend go to the school and tell the principal I was sick. If I wasn't physically ill, I was surely sick of no electricity, boiled water, bad or no food, and the hard work that was my life.

On this day, I found hope in the fact that nothing could go wrong. It was winter or at least as wintry as it gets in the Sahara. Staying inside my mud house was almost pleasant after I sloshed myself with water from the barrel I kept inside to augment the indoor plumbing. I settled down with a book figuring nothing could possibly go wrong as long as I stayed in my bed.

Never having spent time in any desert, I was unaware

that like in Southern California, it doesn't just rain. No, it pours. Man, it pours! And that is exactly what it did that day. Unlike many houses in Gao, my house did not have the popular corrugated tin roof. Mine was simply a flat mud covering. Not only had no one educated me about the torrential downpours that fell... virtually without warning, but no one had advised me of something called... the life span of houses.

My house, like most in Gao, was built of mud bricks mixed with straw and dung. Yes, building season was less than pleasant to the olfactory nerves, but after they dried, these bricks made sturdy houses. After the rain, I discovered another helpful fact about mud houses; they last about five years. I also learned another critical piece of information; the weight of the water on a five-year-old roof can cause a collapse, and since it seems my house was five years old, that's exactly what happened.

As I lay in my bed, secure in the hope that nothing could go wrong if I didn't venture outside, the roof fell on my face. Literally. I was covered in mud, straw and dung as the downpour continued. Now I can laugh, but then, being naked, wet and smelly in the midst of a downpour did not make me happy or hopeful.

Sometimes we place our hope in things we simply cannot control, and despite our best efforts, our world caves in around us. Though I am hopeful for a cure, I prefer placing my hope in getting the best care for my husband. Others hope their children will never get HD, so they adopt theirs to run a better risk of the HD chain being broken. Buying long term and nursing home insurance shows one is placing hope in companies who can help provide for financial needs in the event there is no cure in time. The list of places where people place their hopes is long and unique.

We find hope in small everyday ways, and sometimes, it is exactly enough to get us through one more day. Mary's daughter, Annette, was diagnosed with HD last year. "Hope is sometimes Annette's dimple, when she is really amused at something silly I have done. Today, hope was the gentle rain that my poor flowers needed so badly, and, on Sunday, it was sitting very still in church, surrounded by the certainty that all was well with my soul."

Bonita finds hope in the fact that there is always tomorrow, and tomorrow lives in her precious grandchildren. One of my favorite comments on hope was shared by my friend Ginny who has a daughter with juvenile HD. "Hope comes from looking at the love in my sons' eyes and knowing that we are one with Pam, joined by the thread of love and that her life goes on through us."

To wish for something with the expectation of its fulfillment is to hope. Hope can also be defined as the desire and search for a future good. Whatever its source, we all need it in our lives. The original poem was written about cancer, but I have used Huntington's instead. The author is unknown, but for those who have HD, the words ring with truth, and yes, hope.

∽

What Huntington's Cannot Do
AUTHOR UNKNOWN

Huntington's is so limited
It cannot cripple love
It cannot shatter hope
It cannot corrode faith
It cannot destroy peace

It cannot kill friendship
It cannot suppress memories
It cannot silence courage
It cannot invade the soul
It cannot steal eternal life
It cannot conquer the spirit.

In its most logical form, hope could really be thought of as a defense mechanism that the human mind is equipped with to face overwhelming situations. But whether it is a defense mechanism or not, we all need hope in one form or another – because when all is said, hope is our last line of defense in the face of adversity. Without hope, all that is left is despair.

∽

He Gave Us Today
BY SHIRLEY PROCELL

No promise of tomorrow
He gave us today
That's why it's a gift
Or, so some folks say
You must cherish the moment
Fill the hours with love
Live the day to the fullest
And thank God up above
He gave us today
What more could we ask?
Let us live it as though
It's the best and the last.

Reflections

Anonymous

Darkness fills the room. The moonlight casts shadows on the walls. The clock reads 2:34 a.m. It is always at this time that the thoughts fill my head. During the day, when it is bright and sunny, it is so easy to forget, to pretend that it doesn't exist. But here, with him laying beside me, breathing rhythmically, the sound of his heart beating in my ear, I wonder how I could go on if I lost him. My husband, my best friend, is at risk for having Huntington's Disease. It took me a long time before I could admit that, much less say it. Now the words come more easily. It's only the words that come easily, though. My ideal life includes lots of children, a house with a white picket fence, a few dogs, and a sports utility vehicle, the nineties version of the station wagon. We plan to have it all. But, I would give every bit of that up in half a second for the guarantee that he is HD free. We've come a long way since that very first time I looked up Huntington's Disease in the medical dictionary. At the time, what struck me were the phrases "middle age," "hereditary," and "always leads to death." And with that, my world began spinning. But you pick yourself up and move on. I love my husband more than these mere words can express. He is a part of me and I will stand by him and with him in "sickness and in health." He may get HD; he may not. Either way, I don't regret being with him. In all honesty, if we had known about the HD when we first met, I don't know for sure whether or not I would have gotten involved with him... you know, way back when I barely knew him and certainly did not yet love him. But we didn't know, and I fell in love with him. I haven't regretted it for one single minute.

It's 3:47 now. I hear a dog barking in the distance. The moon has fallen further in the sky. It casts an eerie, blue light across the bed. I look at his face, that precious face. I wonder how he would look; would he lose that sparkle? Would the world look different through his eyes? Would I? I shake my head, trying to clear my thoughts. But they don't go. They're always there, lurking. He's told me that he wouldn't blame me or be angry with me if I decided to leave him and this situation, but I could never do that. He's told me that if he ever gets as sick as his mother is now, he wants me to move on... maybe find someone that could take care of me. How ridiculous! He says these things merely to give me a way out, but he knows I would never go. Sometimes I want to go to the top of a mountain and cry and scream with all my heart and soul that it's just not fair. I don't wish to scream those words for myself, but rather, for my husband. However, we all know that life is not fair. I wipe a tear off my cheek and watch him sleep. There are days when I am totally convinced that he will have HD, but there are weeks when I am certain that he won't. He chooses not to be tested now. I can live without knowing. At least we can hold on to that glimmer of hope that all will be well. I refuse to look for signs and symptoms in everything he does. Life doesn't offer any guarantees for him or for anyone else. For now he takes a lot of pictures... he says it's so I won't forget a single moment. He writes me long letters... he says it's so I'll always remember how much he loves me. He films miles of video... he says it's so I'll always remember how full of life he is right now. Most of all, like everyone else whose lives have crossed paths with this terrible disease, we pray together each night for a cure and the strength to handle what is sent our way. Before I close my eyes, I hear my mother-in-law's voice in my mind. It seems so long ago.

She said, "Please don't be afraid of this. Life is too short for fear." To all my friends... live each day to the fullest... filled with love, light, and laughter. Remember that the angels are watching over all of us.

$$\backsim$$

Where There is Hope

BY GARY

I'm thirty-two years old, and had gone through all the counseling in anticipation of finding out the results of my test. I was even optimistic about receiving the results; I got the shock of my life when they were positive. I think looking for symptoms is a waste of time. While it is important to prepare for the future with insurance and financial planning, one should live as if HD isn't there. If you let the worrying of, "When is it going to hit me?" take over, if you continue to think, "Does that stumble mean it's here?" ...then you are letting HD win twice. It wins once when you get it, and once when it destroys your life until that point.

I won't say that in the back of my mind I don't worry about this thing or that, but the amazing thing is, most people can find one or more symptoms of HD in themselves even though they don't have the gene. Don't worry, because when the symptoms are visible enough, you and those around you will know. Until then, live your life to the fullest. It isn't easy, you say. Right! But you have no choice. Whether you have a spouse and children, other family members or just people who care, don't make things worse for them when it isn't relevant.

I am filled with hope, though some would question the basis for my hope. Amazingly enough, getting the "wrong" answer didn't stop me from looking for the "right girl" and I think I have managed to find her. She apparently cares enough for me to go forward with me, despite the fears, and despite her family's great misgivings. Now does that sound as if I'm giving up already? I will fight HD now and I will fight in the future.

∽

Hope for Carolyn
BY NOEL CROWSON

How can I give hope to my beautiful wife, Carolyn? We are still setting future goals together and I include her in all our planning. If her condition becomes such that she isn't able to handle complex planning or goal setting, then I will set simpler goals that will allow for self-accomplishment with a feeling of self-worth. My years in the military have shown me that men will die for a piece of colored cloth. A pat on the back, a word of encouragement will move mountains. My hope is to provide Carolyn with the best life possible under the worst of situations.

I will shout it from the roof tops if it will help those in need. Huntington's is becoming a fight that I expect to see won in our lifetime. Education is the key. God is also a part of our lives. I see God at work all around me in every rock, tree, person, thought, word or deed. Our God loves everyone and expects us to express His love through service to others. Our major life goal in all our travels with the military has been to never meet a stranger, and always leave friends. Carolyn is the richest person I know, for she has more friends than anyone else I know. She also is my best friend. She has always drawn others to her and has such a sweet nature that people always open up to her. She is one of God's Angels. She makes people feel good about themselves and never mentions any of her problems. As I work to give hope to Carolyn, I realize that in Carolyn, I find hope.

With My Feet Beneath Me

BY GABRIELLE HAMILTON

With my feet beneath me
I experience
    as though each day were all that mattered
and each encounter were worthy of reflection

With my feet beneath me
I live
    with my subconscious soaked in history
and my conscious hungry for tomorrow.

With my feet beneath me
I climb
    on the shoulders of those before me
and the support of those who love me.

With my feet beneath me
I am uncertain
    if I am blinded by the light
or in the darkness

With my feet beneath me
I reach
    for another who,
by reaching for me, finds strength.

With my feet beneath me
I know
    that no matter where I'm going
I will get there.

November 1994

...Just For One More Day

BY JEAN ELIZABETH MILLER

The overwhelming feeling of wanting to bawl your eyes out never leaves you and hits you at the most unexpected times. Fortunately, it's mostly when you're alone with your own thoughts and reality. You can't put your finger on the "one" thing which prompted that reaction; it's not one thing. It's several built up ones. It's something, right now, no one can "make better," and you're weakened by your own sense of not having control.

For those of us who have always commandeered our lives, to suddenly be in a boat without a rudder is more than a little bit scary. Caregiver, affected person, at-risk, it truly matters not. The feeling is the same with moments of total helplessness, abandonment and fear, the unknown, the swelling of the tears.

But then there is our loved one; a child, a wife, a husband, a friend. A special look, a smile, a tender word or two help carry us through to face another battle. It is then that we, who come to this disease from different ends, come together as one. Hopefully, then, our hearts forgive us and we are given the strength to go forward... just for one more day.

As caregiver, at-risk, someone affected, the one and only thing we can do in this disease is to take each and every day one at a time. Today, appreciate, savor and find delight in as much as you humanly can, for as the saying goes, none of us truly knows what tomorrow will bring. If we allow our minds to travel too far into the future, over which we have no real control, we only lose the precious seconds given to us today.

Huntington's Disease: Friend or Foe
BY ROBERTA BRINK

I first learned of Huntington's Disease in my family when I was fifteen years old. My father found out from my grandpa, my mom's dad, when one of my cousins shot himself. Presumably, it was because he thought he carried "the curse." Sadly, he didn't. My mother had never mentioned it before. My dad thought it was because she didn't want to, but in reality, it was because she wasn't aware of the disease.

I am the youngest of three girls. My oldest sister, Dad, and Grandma, my dad's mom, did a lot of research about the disease, only to discover that there wasn't a whole lot of information. By this time, one of my uncles had developed strange behavior and movements. It was believed that he had Multiple Sclerosis until the family became aware of the existence of HD in the family history. Soon the secret was out. My uncle did, indeed, have Huntington's Disease. It wasn't until just a few years ago that I learned about all the bizarre behavior he exhibited.

Huntington's Disease made a huge impact on me at the impressionable age of fifteen. I watched my uncle and knew that if my mom came down with similar symptoms, I could get the disease. I also knew that I wouldn't know if I had it until I was most likely in my thirties or forties.

Soon I noticed that another one of my uncles had the disease, as well as several other more distant relatives. Scary stuff! That's why, when I was seventeen, and began dating, I was very cautious. Not long after my boyfriend and I started getting serious, I told him that HD was in my family. He had a "so what" attitude about it. He told me he had heart disease in his family, so another disease was no big deal. We got married when we both were fresh out of high school.

Secretly, I had decided not to go to college. I didn't want to waste my parents' money on an education I probably wouldn't be able to use, because the "curse" would get me. I told my parents I wanted to get married instead of going to college.

My maternal instincts were quite strong and I felt I wouldn't be happy unless I had children. But I wanted to have my children while I was young, then they would be older when I came down with the disease. When I miscarried with my first child I was devastated. Fortunately, I became pregnant six weeks later, and had my first son when I was twenty. I had my second son when I was twenty-six.

Ever since I learned HD was in our family, I lived my life in five-year increments. I just knew I was going to be dead by the time I was forty, so I didn't look beyond short-term goals.

I loved every job I had, and I excelled at all of them. I had always wanted to be a lawyer, but felt that would take up too much of my precious life with studying.

My mother was a Huntington's pioneer in Iowa. Once she found out what had afflicted her brothers, she became active doing volunteer work for the Committee to Combat Huntington's Disease. I had always wanted to hide the disease in the closet because I was embarrassed by the behavior and movements of my relatives. But that was not going to happen with Mom as a crusader. She preached Huntington's Disease to anyone and everyone who would listen. She kept saying we needed to educate the public. We couldn't get the funding we needed to help all the families affected by HD unless we got the word out. Gradually, she sold me on the idea; I decided that if you can't beat 'em, you better join 'em.

I became treasurer of the Iowa chapter with my mother as president. After that, she and I got re-elected year after year after year. It was fun working side by side with her and watching and listening to her. She was very compassionate and caring; she helped anyone and everyone who asked.

I remember one tearful night when a new family came to our support group meeting for information. Mom was explaining the disease and answering all questions. There was a lady crying and having such a difficult time handling the news that her parent had the disease. She asked Mom how she coped. My mother and my aunt looked at each other and said, almost in unison, "We cope because we have to. We are still healthy, and it is up to us to care for our loved ones. We are here for you." With that, the lady sobbed on; but she had two comforting shoulders to cry on.

My husband and I started noticing slight movements in Mom when she was forty-eight, but as they didn't seem to get worse, I just rationalized that she had been around so many people with HD that she must have picked up some of their mannerisms.

But we kept a watchful eye on Mom for the next ten years. While she didn't seem to get any worse, she was becoming a little more haphazard about her appearance. Later we would learn she was volunteering for fifteen different non-profit organizations. I just figured she was too tired to care for herself as she had before. Mom loved her eight grandchildren so much and volunteered to have them spend the night with her countless times. She was the apple of their eyes, and they hers. There were times when she would suddenly become irritable, but she kept herself so busy that no one faulted her for that.

In May 1989, Mom suddenly got very ill. She went to the doctor almost every day, but didn't get any better. She collapsed one night and was rushed to the hospital where she underwent emergency surgery. She died that day and so did a part of me. She was the catalyst that kept our family together; it will never be the same without her. My marriage crumbled within a year and a half of her death. I attribute my grieving to that breakup.

At the hospital, we remembered to have Mom's brain sent to the brain bank for Dr. Bird to examine. Also, we wanted to know if she did, indeed, have Huntington's Disease. Sadly, we found out she did.

Now more than ever, I had to know if I carried the gene. The test was still expensive in 1989. My sister and I discussed our need to get tested at great length, and how we each had a hidden agenda if we ever came down with HD. We had both decided that we would commit suicide once our quality of life was not what we wanted it to be. It was such a relief to finally get all of my inner feelings out; it was even more of a relief to find out that my sister felt exactly the same way as I.

When I talked to Dr. Conneally on several occasions and told him of my deep desire to get tested, he had me speak with a colleague of his at Indiana University. She told me I needed to give this serious consideration before I went through with it. She also told me that I should have all my ducks in a row, and to make sure I had all the insurance I could ever want. Then she told me to pay for the test myself instead of turning it over to the insurance company. She really opened my eyes to things that I had not even thought about. I went home from my meeting with her more confused than ever. I wanted the test, but it would be years before I would be able to afford it.

I did begin doing my homework, however, so that I was sure I had all the insurance in place that I needed. That way, when I was able to afford the test, I would be ready to proceed with no delays.

The date, March 23, 1993, will always be etched on my brain. That is the day the National Office of the Huntington's Disease Society of America faxed a press release to me stating that the HD gene had been discovered! The first thing I did was call the man I was dating, then I called my dad. I tried to call my sister too, but she was teaching. When I couldn't contain myself anymore, I tracked her down and had the secretary call her out of class. As soon as I started to tell her , I broke into tears of happiness. Then she started crying. The secretary at the school thought she had gotten bad news! For several minutes we both cried hysterically. What a happy day! Next I called my cousin's wife. My cousin had come down with HD a few years before this and I told her to sit down before I told her. She was ecstatic, as she has two sons who are at-risk.

In November 1995, while I was reading "The Marker," a newsletter put out by the National Office of the Huntington's Disease Society of America, I noticed there was now an Iowa pre-symptomatic testing site for HD. I immediately called the number and learned that testing had become much less expensive once the gene was found. It went down from four thousand to three hundred dollars.

Judy, my genetic counselor, was so kind and understanding. She took down information and set up an appointment for me to come in to talk to her. I was nervous at my first appointment. As she was going through the full history of HD, she mentioned that there was a chapter in Iowa, but that she didn't know much about it. Laughing, I told her I was the chapter's treasurer. We have worked together closely ever since.

I had to have three sessions a month apart before I could get my test results at the fourth session. I told no one, except for my new husband and my boss, that I was going through the testing. Finally, in January, my blood was drawn... and then I waited. The next month was a time of pure hell. I was irritable all the time and had a difficult time concentrating. All I could think about was getting the results of my test. That month seemed like an eternity.

I woke on February 15, 1996, to find that it had snowed and snowed and snowed during the night; worse yet, it was still snowing. I went to work amidst blizzard conditions, determined nothing was going to ruin this day for me. The hour had arrived to leave for my appointment, but blizzard conditions made travel extremely difficult. Fearing I would be late for my appointment, I called Judy to make sure she was going to wait for me. She assured me that she would, but told me I could come in the next day if I wanted. "No!" I shouted into the phone. She giggled a little and said not to worry, she would be waiting.

I had told Judy previously that I had lived my life thinking I had HD, so this would either change my life for the better with a negative result, or just confirm what I already knew. There is no way one can prepare for this accurately. I thought I had, but I found out I was wrong.

Judy showed me my test results. The test was negative. I did not have HD! All I could do was grin and sit there. No jumping up and down. No screams of joy. Nothing. Just a smile and a hug for everyone in the room. All I kept saying was, "I'm okay, I'm okay." Then my foot did a sudden twitch. I looked down at my foot, then looked at Judy and said, "Wow! That happens to everybody, doesn't it? It isn't HD!" I would say it took about a month for it to hit me that I was "okay."

Within minutes of leaving Judy's office, my boss phoned me on my cellular phone with a question that could have waited. When I told him I was okay, he said he knew that I was all along. Then he congratulated me.

The first thing I did when I got back to my office was to call my dad. I decided this was something that deserved face to face consideration, so I just asked him if he was going to be home that night. Dad and I shared tears and hugs. He was very surprised that I had gone through with the test because he had encouraged all three of us not take the test.

The hardest part was calling my sisters. It took me one day to call my oldest sister, and three days to call my middle sister. Not knowing whether or not they were okay made it extremely difficult to tell them my results. My oldest sister went through the testing process immediately after finding out that I had; she also tested negative.

When I went to the HD Convention, I had a difficult time sharing my news with people that I knew had HD, or were at-risk. I had no problem telling unaffected spouses and friends, but I guess I suffered from "survivor's guilt" for several months.

At a support group meeting one night, someone asked me to talk about my feelings after finding out I was okay. As I shared my feelings, I noticed that my cousin's wife started to cry. She told me to never feel bad about being okay; I should cherish the joy of knowing that and rejoice. She was extremely happy I was spared, and so was her husband. That night she helped me accept that I had truly been blessed, and I that should be happy.

Yes, HD is horrible and must be stopped. However, I believe Huntington's Disease is my friend and not my foe. Having this in my family has made me a much stronger, caring and compassionate person. I feel sorry for the people who find it important to criticize or to ridicule the disabled or mentally handicapped, those of a different color or sexual orientation. They are the real losers.

Being involved in helping those with HD has given me

hope and has also helped me to choose my career. I am a consultant and lobbyist, and have become very pro-active in health issues at both the state and national levels. I am hopeful that my efforts, and those of others involved with Huntington's, will make a lasting difference. I wish more people would take the time to share their stories with their Congressmen. They really do listen. It is only when people take the time to share their stories that others can begin to understand, to reach out with a helping hand. And that helping hand is often the beginning of hope.

∾

Is There No End?

BY KELLY ELIZABETH MILLER

Is there no end to this shame?
Is there no end to this pain?
Is there no end to the sorrow?
Will there ever be a better tomorrow?

Is there no end to these lies?
Is there no end to these alibis?
I can't stand going home every day
with you and I fighting in every which way.
Will someone tell me why I lie all the time?
Every day is spent with you on my mind.
You are the greatest thing that ever happened to me.
I pray to God every night that things will turn out all right
for you and for me.

I have hope, you know I do.
There's nothing in this world
I wouldn't do for you.

What is Hope?

BY CAROL FLESSEL

Huntington's is so life-encompassing that, at times, hope is all I have left. I work full time outside the home and I am the only caregiver for my husband who is symptomatic. I also have three adult at-risk children. The future is full of uncertainty, and hope is the only thing that keeps me going some days.

Having hope reminds me of all the things that we do have going for us. I run through my hope list mentally at least once every day, and on bad days, when I am just overwhelmed by the adversity of the whole thing, I run through my list many times.

Hope is:

The medications that they have now, non-existent twenty-five years ago, to help control the inappropriate behavior in my husband, which was never able to be controlled in his father and grandmother. The medications enable him to live at home; his relatives were taken to mental hospitals. This is where twenty-five years of medical research help a new generation to function better with this disease, and offer great hope for their future in the next twenty-five years. There is hope that my children will have access to even better medications that provide comfort and relief to them and their families.

The research that is going on now to find a cure and to find drugs to control the manifestations of the disease brings me tremendous hope. It is the grants that fund this research. It is the research that was done with AIDS and the knowledge derived from it that can be applied to research for HD. It is the scientists who devote their lives and careers to uncovering clues, patterns, genes, cellular functions and other mysteries, trying to unearth the knowledge to conquer this disease. They bring me hope.

Hope lies in the knowledge that all of us have been able to absorb from the media, books, internet capabilities; from our doctors and other health professionals, from the Huntington's conventions and all of the professionals who contribute to it and share their knowledge.

The people who have this disease, who are at-risk for this disease, and those who care for them, make me realize just how much hope there is. The courage and effort and energy that they put into the roles they have been assigned are more than just a glimmer of hope.

The cure, which is, I believe, coming within a generation, and the control, which should be available in ten years, give me hope like never before.

Hope is in the effort and energy to give each other support, to push for funding, to live through today and live for tomorrow. The mountain of energy that we all pull together each day to help us go forward is the ultimate hope, because hope is us.

"What a Wonderful World"

BY BRENDA PARRIS SIBLEY

Things will be better come Spring I know
when all the world is abloom.
Our walks will be long and frequent then
when the garden comes alive and the birds sing a tune.
The garden spot I'm planning there will be
your favorite place, just wait and see.
No more days of sitting in the house;
You and I will be out all the time.
You can walk through the garden or sit on the bench,
and I'll work in the soil, the pleasure's mine.
With flowers abloom all around you,
you'll feel better then.
We will picnic in the garden
on fresh vegetables we've grown;
It will all be more pleasant
than anything you've known.
Yes, though now in the dead of winter,
all will be well come Spring
when the vegetables grow in the garden
and the birds gather round the flowers to sing.

∽ 17

Shana's Story

BY SHANA MARTIN

HUNTINGTON'S Disease has been a major part of my life, all of my life. When I was in the eighth grade, I had to write an essay about my mother. It was nice, printed on some official looking paper. I gave it to her afterwards and it is still hanging in her room. A few years ago, since Mom couldn't really talk, she would get mad and throw things – including drinks. One day, she threw a drink and it splattered on the framed print. Now when I show it to people, they think that others have cried on it when it was read because the splatters look like tears running down the page.

This is what the essay says. "I never really knew you before you got sick, but I had heard a lot about you. You were a straight A student, you were involved in sports, and you had a lot of friends. You also were very beautiful and nice. While doing one of your sports, you met my dad. You were soon married, and a few years later, I was born. When I was about six years old, you started to look and act a little different. We took you to Mayo Clinic in Minnesota. We soon found out that you had a disease called Huntington's Disease. We learned that you would get sick and sicker until we could no longer take care of you, and that's what happened. In January, you moved into Ingleside Nursing Home in Mt. Horeb. Every day I pray for a cure for this terrible disease because I miss you very much. Please don't ever forget, no matter how you act, or how you look, you will always be my mother and I will always love you."

I have never really known my mother except for faint memories of when I was an infant. I was in kindergarten when she was diagnosed with Huntington's Disease. She had never heard of the disease that was to change our lives, because she was adopted as a baby. It was hard growing up; I was confused as to why I couldn't be like other kids, and do all of this neat stuff with my mother. I didn't understand why I was chosen to deal with this.

As her disease progressed, her physical signs became obvious; when people saw me with her, I had to suffer their ridicule. School kids can be very cruel, and I got the worst of it. Children made fun of me every day because I had a retarded, psycho, or freaky mother. Every day I went home and cried. Nobody understood what my mom had and what I was going through. They never wanted to meet my family because they were afraid they would get what my mom had. They would ask me, "Why did your dad marry that thing, and how did she have you?" That hurt a lot. I was embarrassed to be around my mother. To this day, I am unable to forgive those kids because they affected the way I treated my mother in her hard times.

Childhood was hard for me since taking care of my mom was a full time job. At first, things weren't that bad. She would just throw tantrums and get very mad for no reason at all. I guess at that stage as a small child, the scariest thing was that I knew that I might not have a very long life.

As the disease process continued, it got to the point where we couldn't leave her at home alone and I was forced to mature very quickly. I didn't have time to take care of baby dolls like my friends did. Instead, I was in a true "mother" position, taking care of my mom. She was constantly losing her balance and falling. Waking up at night, cleaning the blood out of the carpet and accompanying her to the hospital became a weekly routine. Our family had many hard times putting up with each other. My mom was still able to speak, but some of the things she said were cruel because she didn't really understand what was going on. This would frustrate my dad and I and make us mad at her, but in reality, I now know we were really angry at the disease. It was also hard for me because I didn't have a mother to be my confidante as most of my friends did. I think a mother is the most important part of a little girl's life. All I remember growing up with was the knowledge that "Mommy is very sick."

Back then, gymnastics was the focus of my life. As a kid, no matter what problem I had, I would always feel better at the gym. Those kids didn't make fun of me and I was able to do something that I loved, and at which I excelled. I could be having the worst day of my life, but the second I got into the gym, all of my focus went to gymnastics and my life seemed to be perfect again.

Besides the pain of watching my mom get worse, I couldn't see my friends as much as I wanted. When everyone else was doing things on the weekend, I had to stay home and take care of her. Finally, when we could no longer even leave the house for fear she would hurt herself, we decided to put her into a nursing home. I was quite happy about this; that meant I could finally go out on the weekends and do fun things without having to feel guilty and worry. But that feeling soon changed. Life was different without her in the house; things were scary. It was then that I realized how much I really loved my mom, and how hard it was not to have her around. Sure, she was only a half hour away, but it wasn't the same. She wasn't living in the house anymore. The process was so painful and my dad and I were both depressed; everything in our house reminded us of her and how she used to be. It was sad knowing that she was in a home where she didn't know anybody.

My mom has now been in the home for about three years and she is beginning to adjust. We take her out to eat every week and try to spend some quality time with her. She is at the stage where she can no longer communicate, walk or feed herself. I only wish I could put into words how sad it is seeing this happen to a loved one, especially my own mother.

By the time my mom went into the home, I had many other supportive friends who had matured to the point where they knew that the teasing was wrong. I was focused on gymnastics and logrolling by then and that helped immensely. After a few months, things began to feel a little more normal around the house. This is when I began to discover myself. I was starting high school, and I knew that I needed to start finding some true direction in my life.

I took a health class and realized how interested I was in nutrition and sports. I began focusing much of my time on working out, not only in gymnastics and logrolling, but also cross training, like running and lifting weights.

The emotional and physical strain on me has been tough and is complicated to explain. But even though I've gone through all of this, I have still somehow managed to become a fairly normal teenager. I am a good student and I get almost all A's in school. I get that from my mother since she was a wonderful student.

I am eighteen years old and a senior in high school and I have a lot going for me. I am currently involved in gymnastics, logrolling, pole vaulting, karate, body building, and running. In each one of these things I have a chance to succeed, and that keeps up the excitement in my life. I have a chance at winning at the state uneven bars champion in gymnastics. This summer I became the logrolling world championship in the semi-pro division and I will now move up, with chances to excel in the professional division. I have also been offered the opportunity to perform in lumberjack shows all over the United States, Canada, and Australia. I will be going to Diamond Nationals in Karate this September and competing in the Gold Belt division. With pole vaulting, I not only have a great chance at a full scholarship to the University of Wisconsin in Madison, but there is also a chance I will qualify for the Olympics. I am currently working on a video with my trainer to submit to different fitness modeling agencies. One agent said that I have an excellent chance of being a model for muscle and fitness magazines. I am also currently one of the top sprinters in the city. These are all the opportunities I have opened up for myself just by dedicating my time to the things I love to do.

Yes, I know that my mother is dying, and I know that I might only have a few years left of "quality life" because I am at-risk. These facts are always in the back of my mind, but moping around and trying to get people to feel sorry for me is not going to change reality. Instead, I focus my mind on the things that I love. I'm not saying that I don't ever think about my mother; I think about her all the time and love her more than anything. But I keep my mind off my problems by keeping busy.

Some people rely on other things, such as drugs and drinking, to keep their minds off their problems. I suppose that is one way to deal with a tough life, but in the process, they are also hurting their bodies. I am vehemently opposed to using alcohol and other drugs. I couldn't see myself destroying my body and my future with some illegal substance, not even for a little party over the weekend. There are much safer ways to have fun. I always stay busy, and though I admit that sometimes it can all get a bit stressful at times, it is much better than sitting at home thinking about my problems. I would recommend this to anybody, not just people with HD in their lives, to go out and get involved. You should have very little time where you are sitting around doing nothing and being bored. It not only keeps you from dwelling on your problems, but doing things that you love can help you in many other ways too. Everybody has problems, some worse than others. Of course, I know that even if I blocked them out of my mind they would still exist. But I also can't allow those problems to ruin my life either.

The sad thing is, there is no cure for this disease. Yet. I know scientists around the world are trying to find the cure, but no one knows when this will happen. I have a fifty percent chance of having Huntington's Disease so I may only have a few more years of a "normal" life. At this point, everyone is talking about their futures and what plans they have. I just keep wondering, "Will I have a future?" I want to get married and have a family more than anything. What I don't want is to have my children go through what I have experienced, and I don't want to pass this horrible disease on any further.

Another issue I must face is getting tested. Because of

the discovery of the gene, at age eighteen I will legally be able to get tested. The decision of whether to test or not is one that I think about often; it will determine the rest of my life. If I get tested and test positive, I will at least know to do the things in life that I have always wanted to do. If I test negative, that will be the biggest relief anyone could ever imagine. But if I do test positive, I really have no clue how I would handle it. Yet if I don't get tested, I live my life wondering... "Will it happen?" It is a very hard decision and, for now, I don't know what I will do.

Growing up with only my dad has not been easy either. I have no mom to talk to about guys and basic "girl" things. But I really do think that my dad and I have handled our situation to the best of our abilities. We have a wonderful relationship and we have been a support to each other. Through all of this, my dad has never stopped showing how much he loves me. I have learned many valuable lessons. I have learned to live as if each day is my last and that it is precious. We always need to show people that we love them because we never know when it might be too late. Most of all, I pray for a cure.

∾ 18

Faces of Huntington's

BY CARMEN LEAL-POCK

John Quincy Adams is well, but the house in which he lives at the present time has become dilapidated. It's tottering on its foundations. Time and seasons have nearly destroyed it. Its roof is pretty well worn out. Its walls are much shattered and tremble with every wind. I think John Quincy Adams will have to move out of it soon. But he himself is quite well, thank you.

The above is a quotation from John Quincy Adams as he neared death. It was sent to me by a woman afflicted by Huntington's Disease when she heard I was writing this book. How utterly correct are the words when one thinks of those who have, and will die from, the effects of HD. Surely they are tottering on their foundations as the chorea propels them forward. The roof, or the brain, wears out, as does the body. But like Adams, deep inside, those with HD are, themselves, quite well, thank you.

In this last chapter of *Faces of Huntington's*, I have gathered some thoughts that touch on various situations and people who fight the day-to-day battle. Today, as I am writing this chapter, the headlines in newspapers around the world shouted, "Scientists Find How Gene Leads to Huntington's."

It seems that four years after the gene was found, a cure is on the way. For some, a cure could be too late, but their children and grandchildren will benefit. For others just starting their battle, and those not yet born, this gives hope of an incredible kind. If you are a person who is symptomatic or one who is at-risk, there is hope. Have you been tested? There is hope. For caregivers and family members, in the headline you can see hope. Even if it is simply the hope that no one will ever suffer again as have you and yours, it is a wonderful hope.

∼

HD and ME

BY GABRIELLE HAMILTON

You are here
   though you are quiet and
   unassuming at first glance.

You are shy
   though you know me too well
   and are stronger than myself.

You are growing
   with each year though
   you try not to remind me.

You are waiting
   for me to have flown
   before cutting my wings.

I must thank you
   for providing me with a reason
   to live for today.

October 13, 1995

To Ease the Pain

BY LEON JOFFE

To ease the pain I'll use the metaphor of fruit:
Bananas as they rot inside show blackened skin;
Tomato skins reflect the vile decay within;
Yet apples glow with health despite some sickly root.

And so my love, that foul warped seed your fathers sowed
So deeply darkly far inside your beauty's grace
Made not, til now, a single blemish on your face;
Unleashed no inkling of the devastating load

That I, who know it now, must carry hidden far
From you, who also know, that we may live some life.
The apple's rotten core can be expunged by knife,
But every cell contains those genes whose child you are.

And worst of all, the fruit our bodies' seeds have grown:
Our children could be blighted; some; and which unknown.

∾

The Search for an Answer

FROM WRITINGS BY DOREEN GALANTE

"I feel that everybody that comes in contact with HD has a story to tell, of pain, fear, courage, hope and life. It takes a very special person to be able to deal with HD... and an even more special person to be able to do something about it."

—Doreen Galante

May 23, 1997

I guess I'm at a point in my life where I'm asking a lot of questions and I'm not sure where to find the answers. I know there are many situations in the HD community, many not unlike my own. My mother has been afflicted for approximately fifteen years as was her mother before her. I'm the oldest of three and my uncle has it. I've known I was at-risk since I was twenty-three.

As I get older, I've become more fearful of Huntington's Disease. I've managed to enjoy my life in many ways in spite of the trials and pains we all know. On the outside, I'm active; I dive, camp and love my job. On the inside though, I've crippled my emotional life by not allowing myself to get close in a relationship for fear of having to expose my vulnerabilities. I have recently discovered, through a wonderful therapist, that I've carried a bit of anger within myself, and have kept it locked up nicely, along with lots of the painful stuff that I can't think about for too long. What I've kept locked up is the fear of getting "it" and not being able to live my life. The problem is, I haven't exactly seen myself growing old and I've already cheated myself out of the fullness of life.

I've always thought that testing was a bad choice for me, but I am reconsidering. I guess I'm just wondering if there are any folks out there who can identify with the desire and yet the reluctance to test.

June 22, 1997

I just got back from camping on the Delaware River where I did some thinking, some praying, and some venting to a close friend. I have an appointment for July 18th to get my results. Please keep me in prayer everybody. I feel strong today. I feel that ultimately God is in control, though I am sometimes in fierce disagreement with Him.

That's OK, He can handle it.

I've found that my best defense mechanism is to throw all my energies into my work or my child, and I hope I can keep this up for now. But I know that as the date gets closer, it will become very difficult not to think about it, and I kind of feel like it's my date with the Grim Reaper. I keep turning the appointment card over in my hand and it's such a strange feeling. My date with fate.

As far as my dad is concerned, I know he loves me. But going through the whole ordeal with my mother has taken a terrible toll on his health and he has grown weak emotionally. I just have to learn to deal with it, the way I had to learn to accept my mother's inabilities, though I now understand and forgive her and know it's not her fault.

What else can I do now? I've talked for months to my therapist, I've cried, I've laughed, I've cursed God, and asked forgiveness. I've been angry, sad, depressed, and afraid. I've denied, accepted, bargained, pleaded and tried to make deals with God. I've been strong, brave, in charge, and now I feel like the little girl who needs a hug.

July 17, 1997

Tomorrow's the day. Though I've been handling it pretty well for the most part, I think today I can already feel that it's going to be a tough one. I am so nervous that I am trying to take deep breaths and control my thoughts from overtaking me with fear. I've prepared as best as I can for the results, and my support team has been calling me. Everyone thinks I'm going to be fine, which is great. But as I sat in my therapist's office to prepare for the last time, I asked him if I really was ready and he said I'm as ready as I can be. Even though I can work through a good result in my mind, and really can't walk through a bad result, he says that if it should happen, we will work together. He better be ready, because he'll have some major work ahead of him.

God, I've got to get through this day. It's funny, but as I've been talking to people this past week or so, it seems that anything they tell me about their own lives just doesn't matter. If someone talks about their kid's new job, their latest home improvement, the weather, or anything, I've just looked at them and said, "I really don't care about that right now." The ones that know about the test have laughed. I probably won't have too many friends left after this! The point is that nothing else matters and everything else seems trivial. That's not normally my nature, but then again, tomorrow I find out the most important piece of information of my life.

I had a really long talk with my dad the other night and he said he hadn't brought the test up because he didn't want to focus on it. I let him have it and told him that I needed for him to bring it up. He needed to talk about it, not to give me any magical answers, but to show that he cared. We talked for a long while, and it was very healing. I found myself asking him why he married my mother. Funny, but I couldn't believe those words came out of my mouth, and I wonder if somehow, subconsciously, I projected blame to him for HD because I can't blame my mother directly. Anyway, I do love him dearly and I've been giving him a bit of a hard time lately.

I'm quite full of emotion right now, and so many people have expressed their support. I am asking for prayer because today, I really think I'm going to need it.

July 18, 1997

These are more ravings from a crazed lady who has been up again since 5:15 a.m., who can't sleep and feels the need to vent again.

I have butterflies in my stomach and can hardly breathe. Yesterday was a day I shall never forget. Friends far and wide called me to wish me well. Some even cried and much love came my way. Yesterday was like I was in a trance. I was calm, but felt as if my life was flashing before my eyes all day long. I kissed my little one on the head and left her with the sitter overnight because I didn't want her to be around during the night before. As I kissed her, I almost cried because I knew that the next time I saw her I would be a different person; either free in spirit and mind, or extremely upset and depressed. I left my job knowing that there, too, I would return a different person. I saw my dad and brother and knew the same. My younger brother kept looking at me and didn't know quite what to say. All I kept thinking was that I am the strong one in the family, they need me and I have to be okay.

My dearest friend of sixteen years slept over last night and we talked until midnight. All I kept coming back to was a lifetime of being affected by HD and a lifetime of overcoming these effects. I know that I am strong and will deal with whatever comes my way, but I need to know that it is finished. We've gone through so much that I told my friend I just cannot bear to have this. I don't know if anyone can actually be totally "ready" for being told that one has this gene. I am as ready as I am going to be.

July 18, 1997

After a night of hell and this morning crying, praying and driving to the facility feeling like I was walking the "death row walk," I arrived early. I could barely breathe and I just paced the hallway like a caged lion.

The geneticist called me in and I held my dear friend's hand and he gave me my results. I am okay!

I shouted and cried and gave thanks to God and felt all of the anger just melt away. Then I called my father and while I was sobbing, I told him I was okay. He took the sobbing as a bad result and he started to cry. I said, "No! I'm okay!! I don't have the gene!" Then he laughed and cried and told me that he just lost ten years off his life from that scare.

Funny, the sky seems bluer, the trees fuller, the grass seems greener and life has begun anew for me today. I feel like I was born again today and I am so thankful to God, and to all who prayed for me.

∽

Relieved

BY GABRIELLE HAMILTON

I was relieved
that it was over.
Relieved that I now knew
what others had tried to guess,
even me.
Relief has come
despite the anger and sorrow
knowing brought with it.
Relief at ending the guessing games
and furtive attempts
of planning a future.
Relief that I am now firm and certain,
focused and determined
because I know.

Purposeful Ambiguity

BY MARY PRICE

Years ago, I had a Systems Analysis professor who coined the term "purposeful ambiguity" in connection with a caveat about not over-analyzing a situation. He was suggesting that some ambiguity can, and should be, tolerated more often than we sometimes like to admit. That term or concept has become a favorite of mine, and again I draw upon it as I contemplate the results of my HD predictive testing.

On December 4th, I had my last pre-testing counseling session and made my decision to proceed with the blood test. The test results are now in and available; however, I have decided not to be told at this time. That was always an option, but only as a result of the counseling sessions did it emerge to be the right option for me right now.

Given this situation, did I truly learn anything as a result of going through this process? Most definitely, yes, I did. The counseling sessions reminded me that there are many valid reasons for knowing the test results. Very few of them apply to me since I have no children and since, fortunately, I am not facing any life decisions that would be influenced one way or another by the test outcome.

I learned more about "Survivor's Guilt" and realized that I am already having to deal with this as friends in my cancer support group are beginning to die.

Going through the counseling process confirmed that it was very important for me to come to closure on the testing process. Therefore, by going through the pre-testing counseling, having the blood test performed, and having the results stored in a secure and confidential manner, I feel that I have satisfactorily come to closure on the testing process.

Going through the counseling process also confirmed for me that I had a very strong need to know whether or not I had the genetic condition that might lead to HD. I also realized, for the first time, that I had an equally strong need to keep all my options open, recognizing that once I'm told the results, that knowledge cannot be undone. As long as I don't know, I still have the option to know or not know.

Then I had to try to balance two somewhat conflicting needs; the need to know and the need to keep my options open. Having come to closure on the testing process, the decision to know or to not know is now mine. It is no longer a case of not knowing because I can't know or because I'm not allowed to know. I discovered that it is relatively easy to live with not knowing, when it is as a result of my own decision, and not some outside condition beyond my control that prevents me from knowing.

And so I find it quite comfortable at the moment to have this purposeful ambiguity as a part of my life. I recognize that my options are still open, that while I might still have an unfulfilled need to know, it is of my own doing and can be revisited if I change my mind in the future. I have to credit the doctors and staff at Johns Hopkins, for without their good efforts, I never would have come to this position. I must admit that for the first time since HD reared its ugly head in our family, I'm remarkably at peace with my own situation. I feel much more confident in my own abilities to deal with this ambiguity.

Peace of Mind

BY JASPER SWART

She walks and talks differently,
She doesn't move steadily,
I wonder what those people think
When they see her act like that.

She doesn't seem to feel disturbed
By all that's happening to her,
But when we're walking side by side
This burning pain is hard to hide.

Oh mama, what the hell is happening to you?
A big black hole is growing in your mind,
Someday it's going to happen to me too.
A peace of mind is hard to find

There are times when I feel cold
And I'm afraid of growing old,
That's when I need someone to understand
The things I cannot comprehend.

I really long to meet the one
Who will shine on me like a sun,
To keep me warm all through the night
When I feel this fear inside.

Oh darling, when will it happen to me too?
That same black hole will be growing in my mind.
That's when I'm going to need a little help from you,
A peace of mind is hard to find.

An End to Secrecy

BY SHIRLEY C.

How ironic this is! I'm writing this story about the negative effects of keeping Huntington's Disease a secret, yet I'm not signing my last name. Some families keep silent because of shame, or fear. But these aren't my reasons. Out of respect to certain members of my husband's family who have perpetuated the secret, I've chosen this course, too. To stay angry about the secret hurts no one but me, and I've forgiven the secret-keepers; I've accepted the fact that, at the time, they believed they were doing the right thing. I hope my story helps even one person to recognize the importance of honesty when dealing with HD.

When I married my husband in 1979, there were two big family secrets. One was that his oldest sister had a different father than he and his "full" siblings. It seems his mother had been married to another man for just a few months. The second secret was about the mysterious circumstances regarding his birth father's death. The only thing I knew about the death of my husband's biological father in 1971 was that the cause of death was listed as "smoke inhalation."

I knew he'd been in some kind of hospital and had gotten a pass to visit a friend. The night he visited the friend, the rest of the household had left to continue partying elsewhere, leaving him alone in the house. The couch he'd been resting on caught fire, and his body was found later in the shower, where he had apparently sought refuge from the flames. He didn't call to report the fire, but just ran to the bathroom to escape it. Because it was a neighbor that called 911, an assumption was allowed to perpetuate that he was intoxicated, and not thinking clearly.

I also knew that my husband's father was abandoned by his mother, and he was raised by his grandmother. They say that later his grandmother went crazy; the family had built a fence around her home to keep her from wandering the town. My husband's father had a daughter before marrying my husband's mother, and he remarried after their divorce in 1965, and had one or two more kids before he died. From what I can tell, my husband has two full siblings and at least two or three half siblings.

In the early 1990s, my husband's full sister started acting weird at family gatherings. I asked my husband if he thought she'd become an alcoholic, or was, perhaps, abusing prescription drugs. He later confronted her, and she swore that she was not taking drugs or drinking.

After that, she and her husband avoided family gatherings for a few years. She did call us every few months to keep up with the family news, but wouldn't share anything personal herself. As her speech was gradually becoming more and more slurred, my husband and I convinced ourselves that she hid some sort of an addiction. I'm embarrassed to admit that we stopped initiating any kind of contact, although we were polite and loving when she called us.

In March of 1994, my husband's mother passed away from pancreatic cancer. There was a huge family gathering for her funeral, and conversations were stilted and abrupt. I attributed it to grief, but I later learned that other things were brewing.

That summer, my sister-in-law called for a meeting between herself, my husband and me, and their full brother. We built a campfire, and sat up for hours while she told us a horrifying story of her own erratic behavior, the disintegration of her marriage, and of being diagnosed as having either Lou Gehrig's disease or early onset

Alzheimer's. Those were only two of the stories we heard that night. She also wanted to pick our brains about any memories we had about their mother, their real father, or their great-grandmother.

The best information came later, from my husband's stepsister. She admitted that she remembered visiting her crazed step-great-grandparent as a child, and that it was a psychiatric hospital that her stepfather, my husband's natural father, had been a patient in when he died in the fire; he'd been out on pass. My husband and his brother had always been told it was a VA Hospital. They were too young to understand at the time, and the misconception was just never corrected.

The biggest secret didn't come out until the spring of 1995, after my mother-in-law had been dead over a year. It turned out that a few days before she died, she told her sister and her oldest daughter that she suspected that her second husband had Huntington's Disease at the time of his death. She asked these two women to contact my sister-in-law's estranged husband and ask him to try to get her other daughter tested. At this point, my sister-in-law had already endured two years of embarrassing, expensive, and unfruitful tests, and her husband chose to ignore the information as the possible delusions of a dying woman. In 1995, my husband's stepsister produced a packet of correspondence that showed a more than ten-year history of correspondence with, and contributions to, the Huntington's Disease Society of America. It was then that his sister's estranged husband grasped the seriousness of it and began to research the possibility of having her tested. She tested positive in the Spring of 1996, and the first thing she did was call and strongly encourage my husband and his brother to get tested.

The story that both my husband's stepfather and step-sister maintain is that my mother-in-law saw a story in the early 1980s about Huntington's Disease on television. After that, she just decided that her ex had been suffering from HD. They think she felt that if she didn't tell any of her at-risk children about the remote possibility of the gene, they wouldn't come down with it. For my husband, his sister and myself, too many things don't add up. Why the collection of articles on HD and the history of correspondence and contributions? Why did she allow two years of testing her daughter for everything except HD? The final last-minute plea to relatives not at-risk to intervene and get my sister-in-law tested tells a story that has created a huge amount of anger and mistrust within the family. My sister-in-law tried to obtain her father's medical records in 1996, even going as far as obtaining a court order. But the records were either destroyed or filed under a misspelling of the last name.

A long, long conversation between my husband's ex brother-in-law and myself, in early 1996, had me floored. All the crazy and hurtful things my husband had been doing were exactly the reasons their marriage had failed in 1994. I was convinced by the end of the conversation that my husband had HD. The long process that resulted in his ultimate diagnosis in August of 1996 was, for me, just a frustrating and expensive formality. My anger at his family was probably, in part, a result of my anger at the disease, but it was also anger at the secret.

It is easy to see, especially in retrospect, that HD was the contributing cause of my husband's great-grandmother's and father's deaths; and possibly a contributing factor in his grandmother's abandonment of her son.

Because of the secret, I have three at-risk children, although to be truly honest, had I known I probably would have had them anyway. My sister-in-law's marriage has collapsed.

Would their marriage have been saved if her husband had known there was a physical explanation for her actions? Or if she'd been started on the right medication sooner to modify her behavior? Maybe. The family is in turmoil, and trust between step-siblings has been destroyed. Because of these and other family secrets, my husband has a half-sister out there somewhere that may be going through all kinds of tests because she cannot be located and informed. He also has one or two younger half-siblings with potential time bombs ticking inside their bodies.

What am I doing instead of keeping secrets? My three teenage children have been informed since just after my sister-in-law got her positive results. I talk regularly to my husband's brother, who can't afford to get tested, about the early symptoms I noticed.

My brother-in-law, who cannot afford testing, is now forty-five and symptom-free, while my husband's symptoms started in his mid-thirties and his sister's in her late thirties. My kids and I surf the Internet for information on HD. They know exactly how to go about stopping the disease, in this family, in this generation, by choosing to have HD free children. My kids are very open about HD with their friends, and enjoy the support that honesty usually brings. My sixteen-and-a-half-year-old daughter has started the process to be tested as a minor. She wants to plan her future in a realistic manner, and be cautious when she chooses to have kids.

There is one appropriate time for secrecy in HD. Before he was tested, we beefed up all of our life and health insurance policies. We told the absolute truth on all applications, and were turned down only for the nursing home policy. My three kids also have life insurance policies, with guarantees for options to double the coverage at age eighteen and again at age twenty-five, regardless of (their) health. Laws are being changed to stop genetic discrimination in some forms of insurance, but it is still better for an at-risk person to make sure their insurance is as good as possible before beginning any treatment, taking any medication, or being tested.

I read a statistic that said that three in one hundred thousand people have, or are at-risk for HD. Without knowledge, that number could increase to one in ten thousand in one generation and one in one thousand in two generations. The gene is always dominant. Each child of an affected parent has a fifty-fifty chance of carrying the disease. The disease always penetrates. This means that every person who carries the gene will at some point come down with the symptoms.

It is only by stopping the secrecy that this disease can be stopped. It is only by stopping the secrecy that society can begin to understand and accept the victims of this disease.

Lies

BY GABRIELLE HAMILTON

You believed that lie
    without knowing
    or asking
anyone of anything,
as though you made it up
    to make yourself feel better.

I wonder how you felt
    when you were told
    that you too were in jeopardy.
Did you cry?
    Were you in shock?
Or did you feel relief
    at letting go of the lies
    which had separated you
from us?

Your pain is so different
    from mine
as we were shaped
    by different goals and expectations
and yet,
    we are the same.

March 27, 1995

Walking on Life's Fence

BY PAMELA FOYE

It engulfs my life
It affects my world
Even while I am healthy
it rages in a cave just waiting to strike.

Will it strike me
or my younger brother?
Neither or both of us?
What cards has fate dealt?

We see what it does to our mother,
Will that be us soon?
Will that time bomb
ignite in our brains, too?

We are walking on life's fence
which way will we fall?
it has already been decided
thus, with dignity we must accept it...

...in the meantime we must cure HD.

Growing Old Fast

BY BRENDA PARRIS SIBLEY

At forty she looked older,
walked with a shuffle,
an unsteady gait.
By forty-five she had to stop
driving. She said, "If I could
just get my head straight."
By fifty she couldn't live alone.
Her children passed her
around, one by one.
By fifty-five she was in a
nursing home, like an old
woman. Where has time gone?

Copyright © 1997

Lou Wilkinson has begun giving talks to Canadian support groups on what it is like being a person with HD. She was a teacher and is an articulate, witty, wise individual. Her insight into this disease is helping others to better understand their pHD.

At a recent meeting, she made the following statement. "The primary caregiver is the person with HD themselves." She went on to explain that caregivers are actually care partners. "They are not here to be our nursemaids and do not have psychic abilities. Not only that, our care partners have a life of their own and have a right to have that life."

Lou points out a caregiver has rights, but so do persons who have this disease.

A Caregiver's Bill of Rights
AUTHOR UNKNOWN

I have the right...

To take care of myself. This is not an act of selfishness. It will give me the capability of taking better care of my loved one.

To seek help from others even though my relatives may object. I recognize the limits of my own endurance and strength.

To maintain facets of my own life that do not include the person I care for, just as I would if he or she were healthy. I know that I do everything that I reasonably can for this person, and I have the right to do some things just for myself.

To get angry, be depressed, and express other difficult feelings occasionally.
To reject any attempts by my loved one, either conscious or unconscious, to manipulate me through guilt, and/or depression.

To receive consideration, affection, forgiveness, and acceptance for what I do from my loved one, for as long as I offer these qualities in return.

To take pride in what I am accomplishing and to applaud the courage it has sometimes taken to meet the needs of my loved one.

To protect my individuality and my right to make a life for myself that will sustain me in the time when my loved one no longer needs my full time help.

To expect and demand that, as new strides are made in finding resources to aid physically and mentally impaired persons in our country, similar strides will be made towards aiding and supporting caregivers.

To be myself...

᭤

A pHD's Bill of Rights
BY LOU WILKINSON

A person with HD has the right...

To be treated with respect.
To have it recognized that they are doing their best.
To have it remembered that they may not be aware
      of their behavior.
To be allowed to take extra time to understand
      what is being said or expected.
To have fun, to dance, to try to make jokes.
To receive patience rather than scorn when trying to
      do something or remember something.
To have a life that isn't dictated one hundred percent by
      their caregiver.
To be forgiven for forgetfulness, clumsiness and
      lack of focus.

Alternative Stages of Huntington's Disease

BY JIM POLLARD AND ROSEMARY BEST

Defiance:

"I'm not denying the diagnosis, I'm defying the verdict! I'm not refusing to accept it, I'm just boldly resisting the inevitable!"

Perseverance:

"I'm continuing on... in spite of all the difficulties this disease puts in front of me."

Compassion:

"I'm sorry for the trouble I'm causing my family and everyone else who cares for me. I wish I could do something to help them."

Stamina:

"I'm not sure just what it is but something keeps me going! It keeps me going through all my fatigue and all the problems and hardship this disease presents me."

Grace:

"I've quietly resigned myself to needing others to care for me, to sustain me. I can't show them, but I'm more concerned for the welfare of those around me than I am for myself. We know we're there for each other."

A Brand New Day

BY SHIRLEY PROCELL

As the sun came up
On a brand new day
The sky was brighter
Or it seemed that way
For with the dawn
Came new courage and hope
The thread we hung on
Has become a rope
We can believe in time
That a cure will be
Or at least some help
For those with HD
So send up the prayers
On this brand new day
So that good news
Can continue our way.

Appendix

I N *Faces of Huntington's,* I have specifically left out medical terminology and facts about Huntington's Disease. I am not a physician and the purpose of this book is to address the people side of the disease. While this is not a complete listing, there are many excellent resources available. In addition to these listed, there are also a number of booklets on a wide range of topics, a number of which are free or can be ordered for a nominal fee. All these resources can be obtained through the Huntington's Disease Society Association by calling 1-800-345-HDSA.

Brain and Blood Donations

The donation of a brain or blood from a person with HD is a tremendous gift of hope to research and future generations. For more information on brain tissue donation write or call:

Harvard Brain Tissue Resource Center
McLean Hospital, 115 Mill Street
Belmont, MA 02178-9106
(800) 272-4622

Dr. Wallace W. Tourelotte, Director
National Neurological Research Bank
West Los Angeles VA Medical Center
11301 Wilshire Blvd.
Los Angeles, CA 90073
(310) 268-3536

To bank blood samples call or write:

Bank by Mail Program
National HD Roster Project
Indiana University Medical Center
975 West Walnut Street
Indianapolis, IN 46202-5251
Call collect: General: (317) 274-2241
DNA Bank: (317) 274-5745
HD Roster: (317) 274-5744

Resources on Huntington's Disease

Understanding Huntington's Disease: A Resource for Families.
Huntington Society of America, 1997, 48 pages (previously published by Huntington's Society of Canada). This
informative booklet is divided into three sections: Facts
About HD, which covers symptoms, diagnosis, preva-
lence, treatment, and genetic testing; Experiences of Family Members; and Living With HD, which includes coping

with being at-risk, marriage and parenthood, counseling, and therapeutic interventions.

Genetic Testing for Huntington's Disease: A Guide for Families, HDSA, 1996, 18-page booklet. An introductory guide to genetic testing for HD in question and answer format.

Caregiving Packet (includes the following):
Practical Hints for Caregivers, HDSA, 1988, 9 pages. Covers eating, swallowing, clothing, cleanliness, communication, smoking, recreation and attitudes.

Westphal, Beryl. 1995, *Nursing Tips: A Collection of Caregiving Hints*, HDSA, 9 pages. A compilation of professional caregivers' suggestions on feeding, communication, behavior and other daily concerns.

Dird, Edward et. al. 1984, *Huntington's Disease Management*, Middlesex County Hospital, MA, 6 pages. Dressing aids, relaxation, nutrition, communication, physical fitness.

Chiu, Edmund. 1991, *Caring For Persons With Huntington's Disease. 2nd edition.* New York: Huntington's Disease Society of America, 150 pages.

Elliott, Wendy. 1993, *Living with Juvenile Huntington's Disease.* Huntington Society of Canada, 67 pages.

Greene, Rickey. 1992, *You Are Not Alone: A Guide to Establishing Huntington's Disease Support Groups.* HDSA, New York, 56 pages.

Ranen, Neal G. 1993, *A Physician's Guide To The Management of Huntington's Disease: Pharmacologic and Non-Phar-*

macologic Interventions. New York Huntington's Disease Society of America, 47 pages. Published with funding from the Foundation for the Care and Cure of Huntington's Disease. Includes bibliographical references

Werbel, Eileen. 1990, *Toward a Fuller Life: A Guide To Everyday Living With Huntington's Disease.* New York : Huntington's Disease Society of America, 8 pages. Looseleaf. Published with funding from the Foundation for the Care and Cure of Huntington's Disease. Divided into three sections: Meeting Challenges, Getting Help, How To Cope.

Wexler, Alice. 1995, *Mapping Fate : A Memoir of Family, Fisk, and Genetic Research.* New York: Times Books: Random House, 294 pages. Acclaimed autobiographical account of the Wexler family's personal battle with HD, and their efforts to conquer it by spearheading the research effort.

The Internet provides a wealth of information for those who have access to on-line services. The following is a list of a few available resources. By following links within the pages, you will find a vast array of additional sites that you may find of interest. Please remember, the addresses must be typed in exactly as they appear or you will not be able to access the documents. All links were active at the time of writing.

Electronic Resources on Huntington's Disease

Huntington's Disease Information compiled by Renette Davis. This is an extremely valuable and frequently updated page. Renette welcomes contributions from others and her pages include poems and stories by HD folk and care-

givers as well as up-to-date links to medical information and conference reports. Her bibliography of Huntington's disease resources is an invaluable resource.
http://www.lib.uchicago.edu/~rd13/hd/

Home Page for the Huntington's Disease Society of America.
http://neuro-www2.mgh.harvard.edu/hdsa/hdsamain.nclk

Huntington's Disease Menu maintained by Harvard University Department of Neurology. This page includes information, a message board and the ability to chat with others who are involved with HD.
http://neuro-www.mgh.harvard.edu/forum

An excellent source of information about HD, compiled and maintained by Rob Laycock.
http://www.interlog.com/~rlaycock/2nd.html

Facing Huntington's Disease, a pamphlet published by the Huntington's Disease Association in the U.K. is an excellent source of basic information about all aspects of HD. Thanks are due to the Massachusetts General Hospital and Bill McMenemy for making it available on the web. It is sensitive and straightforward and covers a lot of information beyond the medical facts.
http://neuro-chief-e.mgh.harvard.edu/mcmenemy/facinghd.html

Caring for People with Huntington's Disease. This page from the Kansas University Medical Center Department of Neurology deals primarily with issues of patient care and management. This is a very informative page and includes many links to outside resources too.
http://www.kumc.edu/hospital/huntingtons/

The Hereditary Disease Foundation. The foundation exists to foster and fund research for HD and other hereditary diseases and was founded by Dr. Nancy Wexler.
http://www.hdfoundation.org/

Spanish Language Web Site
http://www.redestb.es/personal/mtor/index.htm

Twenty Steps to Help Caregivers.
 http://www.lib.uchicago.edu/~rd13/hd/steps.html

Hints for Writing to Your Legislator.
http://www.lib.uchicago.edu/~rd13/hd/hints.html

Insurance Strategies for the HD-Affected Family.
http://www.interlog.com/~rlaycock/hd_insur.txt

Mailing List for Huntington's Disease listed in *Faces of Huntington's* as the on-line support group or Hunt-Dis.
http://www.lib.uchicago.edu/~rd13/hd/mailing.html

HDSA Chapter Websites

Georgia Chapter
http://www.akorn.net/~svc/hdsa/

Greater Los Angeles Chapter
http://members.aol.com/hdsala/hdsala.html

Illinois Chapter
http://www.lib.uchicago.edu/~rd13/hd/illinois.html

FACES OF HUNTINGTON'S

Iowa Chapter
http://members.aol.com/rbrink4656/hdsa.html

Massachusetts Chapter
http://neuro-www3.mgh.harvard.edu/hd/hdindex.htm

Mid-Michigan Chapter
http://www.iserv.net/~hdsamich/index.html

Minnesota Chapter
http://www.adverworld.com/id/0015/2105/

New Jersey Chapter
http://members.aol.com/hoopathon/index.html

Northeast Ohio Chapter
http://www.lkwdpl.org/hdsahome.htm

Northern California Chapter
http://ivory.lm.com/~mccarren/n_ca/

Western Pennsylvania Chapter
http://www.telerama.com/~mccarren/winter_96/

HD-related news and events in Canada
http://www.interlog.com/~rlaycock/hscmain.html

Huntington's Society of Canada, Ottawa Chapter.
http://www.comnet.ca/~bfraser/jtmunn/hunthome.htm

South Africa Huntington's Disease Home Page.
http://www3.fast.co.za/~francop/hd0001.htm

Australian Huntington's Disease Association (Vic) Inc.
http://www.vicnet.net.au/~ahda/

There are many HDSA Chapters and Support Groups throughout the United States. A listing of the city and states that have chapters follows. Please call the HDSA office at (212) 242-1968 or 1-800-345-HDSA for more information.

There are currently over one hundred Huntington's Disease support groups. For information on attending an existing group, or starting one in your area, please contact the HDSA office.

Huntington's Disease Society of America Chapters

HDSA Arizona Chapter
Glendale, AZ

HDSA Greater LA Chapter
Beverly Hills, CA

HDSA Northern California
San Ramon, CA

HDSA San Diego Chapter
San Diego, CA

HDSA Rocky Mountain Chapter
Denver, CO

FACES OF HUNTINGTON'S

HDSA Connecticut Chapter
Southington, CT

HDSA Washington Metro Area Chapter
Fairfax, VA

HDSA South Florida
N. Miami, FL

HDSA Georgia Chapter
Decatur, GA

HDSA Idaho Chapter
Coeur d'Alene, ID

HDSA Illinois Chapter
Chicago, IL

HDSA Indiana Chapter
Greenwood, IN

HDSA Iowa Chapter
Orient, IA

HDSA Kentucky Chapter
Louisville, KY

HDSA Maryland Chapter
Baltimore, MD

HDSA Massachusetts Chapter
Boston, MA

HDSA Mid-Michigan Chapter
Lansing, MI

HDSA SE Michigan Chapter
Mt Clemens, MI

HDSA Minnesota Chapter
Minneapolis, MN

HDSA St. Louis Chapter
Webster Groves, MO

HDSA New Jersey Chapter
Cranbury, NJ

HDSA Greater New York-Long Island
New York, NY

HDSA Rochester Chapter
Rochester, NY

HDSA Central Ohio Chapter
Columbus, OH

HDSA Ohio Valley Chapter
Cincinnati, OH

HDSA NE Ohio Chapter
Cleveland, OH

HDSA Oklahoma Chapter
Oklahoma City, OK

FACES OF HUNTINGTON'S

HDSA Delaware Valley Chap
Philadelphia, PA

HDSA Western PA Chapter
Pittsburgh, PA

HDSA Sioux Valley Chapter
Sioux Falls, SD

HDSA Texas Chapter
Bedford, TX

HDSA Northwest Chapter
Seattle, WA

HDSA Wisconsin Chapter
Milwaukee, WI

There are also Chapter Social Workers and Family Services Coordinators in the following states. Please call the national HDSA office at (212) 242-1968 or 1-800-345-HDSA for more information.

Alabama	New Jersey
California	New York
Colorado	Ohio
Georgia	Pennsylvania
Indiana	South Dakota
Kentucky	Texas
Michigan	Wisconsin

Residential Care Facilities

The following care facilities accommodate a relatively high number of people with HD or have a dedicated unit for people with HD.

Edgemoor Geriatric Hospital
9065 Edgemoor Drive
San Diego, CA 92071
(619) 258-3001

Mediplex Skilled Nursing and Rehabilitation Center of Lowell
19 Varnum Street
Lowell, MA 01850
(508) 454-5644

University Good Samaritan Center
22 27th Avenue, S.E.
Minneapolis, MN 55414
(612) 673-6270

JFK Hartwyck at Cedar Brook
1340 Park Avenue
Plainfield, NJ 07068
(908) 754-3100

Terence Cardinal Cooke Health Care Center
1249 Fifth Avenue
New York, NY 10029
(212) 360-3711

FACES OF HUNTINGTON'S

Western State Hospital
P.O. Box 94500
Fort Steilacoom, WA 98494
(509) 582-8900

International Huntington's Disease Associations

Voluntary HD organizations exist in many countries throughout the world. They offer a range of services and care programs to benefit people with HD and their families, and are useful sources of information and referrals for both families and health care professionals. There are chapters in the following countries:

Australia	Netherlands*
Austria	New Zealand
Belgium	Northern Ireland
Canada	Pakistan
Czech Republic	Russia
Denmark	Scotland
England	Slovakia
France	South Africa
Germany	Spain
Ireland	Sweden
Israel	Switzerland
Italy	
Mexico	

*Also the initial contact for organizations in Brazil, Ecuador, Finland, India, Indonesia, Malta, Paraguay, Poland, Romania, Slovakia, Zimbabwe, Tanzania, Saudi Arabia and other African countries.

Contributors

FACES of Huntington's has two types of chapters. Alternating chapters allow you to read someone's story and know how they are affected by Huntington's Disease. However, each of the "Faces" chapters are actually a compilation of essays and poems by several different people. Sometimes, the authors' involvement with HD is not clear through their work. A brief biography of several contributors appears below.

CARMEN LEAL-POCK is the full time caregiver to her husband, David, and the mother of two teenage sons. Prior to this period of her life, she was a marketing consultant and small business owner. Carmen is an author, singer, and speaker and has been a popular presenter at recent HDSA conventions. She has a number of motivational programs using both her speaking and musical abilities. For information about scheduling Carmen for speaking engagements or concerts, call (407) 328-0981. She may also be reached via E-mail at promo@digital.net.

GABRIELLE HAMILTON, MSW, CSW, is the current president of the Greater New York/Long Island Chapter of the Huntington Disease Society of America. Many of her family members have suffered from the disease and she is at-risk for becoming symptomatic. Gabrielle's poetry is featured in several chapters.

LEON JOFFE and his wife, Pitta, are South Africans. Leon is a powerful poet and his work can be found through this book. Three years ago Pitta was positively diagnosed as having HD and is currently in the early phases of the disease. She is an attractive, brilliant woman, recognized as an expert on South Africa's indigenous plants. Her coffee table book, *The Gardener's Guide to South African Plants*, is today regarded as the best book of its type in South Africa. They have four children.

SHIRLEY PROCELL is the mother of two HD positive sons. She has provided endless joy and wisdom through her poetry.

KEN SHEARS is the author of *The City*. He lovingly provides care to his beautiful wife, Rose, who has Huntington's Disease.

HAROLD was diagnosed with Huntington's Disease in 1970 and died in 1986. He was a minister and a musician.

JEAN ELIZABETH MILLER is the mother of Kelly Elizabeth Miller. Kelly has juvenile HD. Jean's poetry touches the heart and can be found in several chapters.

BRENDA PARRIS SIBLEY'S ex-husband's mother has Huntington's Disease. She's in her sixties now and has been in a nursing home for several years. They saw her declining gradually through the years, even before a diagnosis was made. She knows the fear that her ex-husband and his brothers and sisters have, that they, too, may have this disease. She personally knows a similar fear now, because her mother had Alzheimer's Disease, and she fears growing old and having it herself.

MONTSE TORRECILLA lives in Barcelona, Spain. She is active in the Huntington's Disease Association in Spain, and is in the process of translating web pages into Spanish along with maintaining her own HD web site.

THE AUTHOR OF "TO MY SISTER" tested negative for HD almost two years ago. She is the oldest of three girls born to a father affected with HD. During her father's final years, her middle sister developed juvenile HD. Her youngest sister and she have always clung together.

CHRISTOPHER KLINE is owner/director of chc associates casting and services, a casting and production support service for feature film, television and the professional stage. He is a producer/director/actor/writer/designer and is a Nationally Certified Educator and State Licensee Examiner. Chris has taken the computer nickname, Uriel, for when he is on Hunt-Dis and other cyber communities. In the Bible, Uriel, meaning Bringer of Light, is actually an archangel, a messenger and protector of the Faith. Chris uses this name because of his desire to spread the good news of God's miracles... a messenger and a bringer of light.

KELLY MILLER is thirty years old and was diagnosed with juvenile HD when she was sixteen. This disease has robbed her of the chance to experience the gifts of life, like independence, the love of a husband, children and lasting friendships. Some of her poems were written in her pre-teens and teens, when she could still hold a pen to write. Kelly is her mother's most profound joy and love in this life and she gives her a great sense of pride. The lessons Kelly teaches people are humility and unselfish love. She finds joy in almost everything, gives from the whole of her heart and forgives all injustices human beings have been capable of inflicting. She is, without any doubt, a beautiful angel on earth.

ELTON HIGG'S daughter, Cynthia, has Huntington's Disease. *The Wild Plant* was written a couple of years ago, when he had a situation with Cynthia. This is a meaningful poem to anyone who has had to deal with a rebellious child.

MARY EDWARDS, author of *Memories of Dad*, is a loving caregiver to her daughter Annette who has HD.

Working with Huntington's Disease in Iowa is a family business. **DIANA FISHER** was Iowa Chapter President from June 1989 to August 1995. She is currently the Family Service Coordinator and Educator, which includes answering the patient service line and teaching in-services to facilities who have HD patients as well as at the Community Colleges. Her husband is the vice-president of the Iowa Chapter, and her sister, **ROBERTA BRINK**, is the current Chapter President.

MURRAY DANIEL THOMPSON is an ardent advocate of persons with Huntington's Disease and lives in Melbourne, Australia. In his quest to help educate others, he is a hero.

BRUCE, the author of *Heart For Any Fate*, lost his mother and aunt to this desperate disease. This psalm was dedicated to them and to his cousin Harvey, who also became a victim of Huntington's Disease. Harvey is survived by his wife and two children. Having turned thirty-nine, Bruce embraces his uncertain future with a heart for any fate.

MARY CHRISTOPHER is a writer living in England. Her husband's father and uncle developed Huntington's Disease, but she shares that she does not believe her husband or children are at-risk, because of what Jesus achieved on the cross of Calvary. She believes that 'By His wounds we are healed' (Isaiah 53:5) and that Jesus heals 'every disease and sickness' (Matthew 9:35).

JASPER SWART is a composer of music for film, lives in Amsterdam in the Netherlands. The poem is actually a song written for his mother who is currently in a nursing home. He tested positive for the gene six years ago but is filled with hope. Last year he married and has faith that there will be a cure soon.

PAMELA FOYE is currently at-risk, actively working as a research assistant in a neuroscience laboratory, and engaged to be married. Because Pam prefers living with ambiguity over a positive test result, she chose not to take the gene test.

Order Form

To order additional copies of *Faces of Huntington's,* please complete the following form (please print):

Name: _____

Address: _____

City: _____ State/Prov: _____

Zip/Postal Code: _____ Telephone: _____

_____ copies @ $15.95US/$21.95Cdn.: $_____

Shipping & Handling: (add $4.00) $_____

Florida residents add 6.5% Sales Tax: $_____

Total amount enclosed: **$**_____

For each copy of *Faces of Huntington's* purchased, $2.00 will be donated to the organization of your choice listed below. Donations will be mailed quarterly.

Please send my donation to:

_____ Huntington's Disease Society of America
_____ Huntington's Society of Canada
_____ Hereditary Disease Foundation
_____ My local chapter or support group (Send to the following address) _____
_____

Volume discounts are available as a fundraiser to associations and chapters. Please enquire for special pricing info. Please send check or money order made payable to:

Living Hope, Inc., P.O. Box 952163, Lake Mary, FL 32795-2163
Send E-mail enquiries to promo@digital.net